FULL CIRCLE

FULL CIRCLE

THE SEGUE FROM ANCIENT CELTIC MEDICINE TO
MODERN-DAY HERBALISM AND THE IMPACT THAT
RELIGION/MYSTICISM/MAGIC HAVE HAD

Laura Veazey

authorHOUSE®

AuthorHouse™
1663 Liberty Drive
Bloomington, IN 47403
www.authorhouse.com
Phone: 1-800-839-8640

Published by AuthorHouse   04/19/2012

ISBN: 978-1-4685-6416-7 (sc)
ISBN: 978-1-4685-6415-0 (hc)
ISBN: 978-1-4685-6414-3 (e)

Library of Congress Control Number: 2012905051

TABLE OF CONTENTS

LIST OF TABLES

LIST OF FIGURES

ACKNOWLEDGEMENTS

There are so many dear ones that I would like to thank for their help, love, and nurturing over the years; those without whom I would not have had the courage to face the struggles inherent in continuing to write and publish.

In 2005, I was told by two (2) male supervisors, that only women pursued EdDs and that few women were bright or accomplished enough to receive PhDs. This presented an immediate challenge to someone already possessing an EdD, and a challenge for which I am truly grateful. Though they were serious in their disdain of EdDs and evidently, women in general, I was determined that I would soon begin work in a field I was quickly falling in love with. Thus began my serious journey into naturopathy.

With every part of my being, I want to thank Peter Allan Childs, my anam cara, for all of his love, nurturing (sometimes prodding), and support. By the grace of God, Allan embraced the challenge for me to write, continuously monitoring my work, and sometimes making it more of a priority than I did. Thank you.

I want to thank my mother, Veazey Groenwold, who taught me at an early age that no matter what, you must get an education and to take chances with those things which are important to you.

My new dad, Heyo Groenewold, now passed, was an incredible source of support, wisdom, kindness, laughter, and love. I only wish that I might have possessed the knowledge to give him a better quality of life during his long bout with five (5) different forms of cancer. I love and miss you past the moon.

I want to thank my dear friend and former committee chairperson, Dr. Janice Martin, who gave me encouragement, direction, and support during this process, encouraging me to publish. You opened new worlds for me. Thank you so very much.

My friend, Mike Taylor, always told me to find my passion and do it. Though he passed a short time ago, his words still ring true and helped to give me the courage to complete this book. This, in part, is dedicated to him.

There is a saying that goes, "friends are your chosen family." If this is so, then I certainly have a very large family. I would like to thank so many, but in particular, the following individuals for all of their love, strength, support (and for some, the music, as well), throughout this long process: Dr. Betty Donohue, Jill and Meghan

Brady, Kami Hoar, Karoly Czinege, Dolores Steward, Cathy Crouch, and Judy Black.

Thank you to each of you for believing in me, for nurturing me, for supporting me, and for loving me. Life gets chaotic enough on its own, and yet, even with my addition to that, you still stood by my side.

PREFACE

Full Circle: A Segue . . .

Consider if you will, what a circle actually is. It has no beginning and it has no end. To come full circle, one has to begin at some point and return again, thus, the segue or bridge, from one point to another. This, then, is what this book is about; the journey from one point of healing to another and how each has impacted the other.

For me personally, this work has been a reflection of much of my own journey; my own quest for answers, both in my personal and professional life and both historic and current. For you see, one typically doesn't write about something unless s/he is somehow invested in it.

My own journey into alternative medicine probably began in the early 1970's, when, as a young teen "hippie," I became fascinated with health food stores and books related to natural health, healing, and childbirth. Having lived on a reservation in my early teens, I was exposed to a lot of folk and Indian medicine. Later, that interest was sparked by the need and desire to help heal a very sick pet.

In 1999, a beautiful St. Bernard puppy, by the name of Mina was born and gifted to my family. Unfortunately, the first owner lied about her having received her shots and she caught Parvo. She died four (4) times and for that veterinarian's aid, I am truly grateful. However, Mina developed a terminal disease and, at the age of nine (9) months, I was told that her immune system had been totally compromised and that, even with the dips and medications, she would have to be put down by the age of two (2). I was determined to find a way to help her and hopefully, prolong her life. At that point in time, I was fairly new to the world of the internet, but began searching for answers. I found topical, temporary relief for her, then began searching for disease cures. Eventually, I found a holistic veterinarian, I know only by the name of "Louise." I had already been learning about herbal remedies and had been using them minimally in my own life. However, Louise walked me through a road of recovery for Mina. Her instruction and Mina's subsequent healing, helped me on my own journey into Naturopathy. I give thanks to both of you. (By the way, Mina is now a 12 year-old pup and aging gracefully).

CHAPTER ONE

The Journey Begins

Modern-day herbalism has its roots in many facets of history. Though herbs have been used medicinally throughout time, I have focused efforts on seven (7) areas of herbal medicine for research, comparison, and contrast:

- Celtic herbal history (inclusive of healers);
- Druidic medicine;
- Native American medicine;
- Christianity;
- Witchcraft;
- Voodoo; and
- 20th and 21st Century herbalism in America, focusing primarily in the South.

I have endeavored to connect each facet, as with a dream catcher, therefore bringing the past to the present. Additionally, the role of magic, religion, and mysticism, and the subsequent impact and influence that they have had through the ages, will be addressed. Through this book, it is hoped that you will articulate why modern-day herbalism has struggled in some instances, and in other instances, has become a successful means of healing.

In the American Indian culture, there is a tool called the Medicine Wheel. It is a circle divided into four (4) segments, with each segment attending to the four (4) components of the human make-up.

The American Indian medicine wheel will be used as a map to guide the research in each facet, thus breaking components into four (4) areas:

- Spiritual;
- Emotional;
- Physical; and
- Intellectual.

Each of these facets has been affected immensely through history and lent a hand to wellness and disease issues. Each facet reveals how each person has been affected by risk factors, thus allowing for unhealthy living skills, then, what communities can do to help alleviate those risk factors and bring the wheel into balance, thus promoting a healthy life circle.

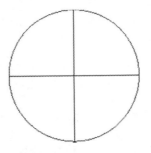

Native American Medicine Wheel

Figure 1A.

Herbalism has been used throughout history, though, for the purposes of this book, focus will begin with Ancient Celtic medicine and move forward to modern-day herbalism. Research will be undertaken to show the degree to which it was/is used, as well as what, if any, impact religion/mysticism/magic has had on herbalism.

Religion, mysticism, and magic have played a significant role in herbalism throughout time. The ancient Celts and druids, in particular, used mysticism and magic as a means of control over individuals.

Druids played an immense role in the lives of Celts and in Celtic society as a whole. In ancient Ireland, druids were broken down into three classes: Bards, Ovates, and actual Druids. A bard (keepers of history; writers, poets, and musicians) could actually make or break an individual through his expertise and opinion in verbal or written prose or song. The Ovate (sorcerers, mystics, and/or healers), was a dangerous one; a soothsayer or seer; one who made potions, devised omens, and attended to rituals and sacrifices. The third class were those who were actually classified as Druids. They were of the highest order of healer, teacher, philosopher, and/or lawyer. They were those who were the keepers of knowledge, history, laws, and traditions. They were given ultimate authority in all matters whether they be sacred or everyday.

The druids held themselves to be even above royalty. In fact, kings throughout history have been known to go nowhere without a druid by their side. Druidic priests have been known to call themselves the creators of the universe, so had been given the ultimate in respect and admiration, coupled with a fair amount of awe and fear.

Their power was incredible and level of knowledge vast. That knowledge was learned over as much as a twenty-year apprenticeship and was passed on and taught by word-of-mouth.

Druids were the keepers of traditional wisdom, thus enabling them to be accomplished in such tasks as dream interpretation and through the interpretation of ritual questions. It also helped in the construction of calendars, which were based on seasonal changes and feast days.

The druidic concern with moral philosophy made the priests very skilled at being judges. As judges, they were tasked with doling out punishments and rewards; the punishments ended many times in human sacrifice. Those sacrifices were sometimes public, an appeasement to the gods, or in private and perhaps as a means of correcting a perceived wrong, such as cowardice in the face of battle. They were typically done for religious and/or spiritual purposes. Some sects even practiced flesh-eating and considered it to be a wholesome remedy for particular ailments.

Celtic healers were both male and female. The Ovates were considered to be the druidic native healers and specialized in healing through the application of natural remedies, and the use of plants, herbs, and trees; working with the four elements; and at times, acting in an ancient version of modern-day psychotherapists.

Wicca is an off-shoot of the Celtic/Druidic tradition. It is based on belief in female deities and has a strong affinity for working with nature and the elements in rituals and healing, as well. Additionally, they believe in the "fey," also known as the faerie-folk.

What is known as American Indian medicine is a combination of both religion and medicine. Plants and herbs have been used to heal and in ceremony for thousands of years. Those plants and herbs have been used ritualistically and with magic and through the use of a medicine man/ woman or medicine priest(ess). The medicine man has been known through many more titles: doctor, man of magic, healer, diviner, and/or person of mystery.

This form of medicine, and in fact, the whole culture and way of life is built around putting one back into balance and harmony. Minor injuries or ailments are typically treated with herbal remedies using the "like cures like" (equated with the Doctrine of Signatures) concept. When there is no relief, the medicine person turns to the supernatural to explain and/or, bring relief.

Voodoo is a religion which began in West Africa, whereupon, slaves took with them to Haiti. It then came to the United States, primarily located in Louisiana. It combines elements of Roman Catholicism, such as having adopted the names of Catholic saints and using some of the Catholic traditions such as prayers, inclusive of the Lord's Prayer, the Hail Mary, baptism, and using the sign of the cross.

Charms, potions, and amulets have many uses; poisons, healing, and protection. Trees, plants, and herbs are used along with other elements to make them. Magic, fear, and superstition are primary tools of a Voodoo priest or priestess.

Modern-day herbalism saw a decline in the 1950's, when an allopathic mentality took hold. Prescriptions of all sorts (ex., antibiotics, diet pills, tranquilizers, etc.) became quick-fixes. However, in the Appalachian region, herbalism and natural healing was and is a continuous part of the culture.

Though a majority of individuals in the area align themselves as Christians, there is a term used to identify the Appalachian culture and that is "Appalachian magic." Many of the original settlers in the area were from Ireland, so much of the magic, superstition, and beliefs came with them and were passed on to future generations. Obviously, the knowledge and use of herbs and plants for healing, potions, charms, and curses was passed on, as well. Faith-healing, witchcraft, snake-religion, Wicca, and Indian medicine are all considered to be bit and part of that culture, even today.

Definition of Terms

Throughout this book, several terms are used to describe terms associated with naturopathy and healing, especially as quoted from existing literature. However, for consistency of language, ease of understanding, and readability within the text, these terms have been employed as they are in conversational language or professional dialogue.

For consistency of interpretation, the following terms are defined as they are used in this research:

Celtic-"A branch of the Indo-European family of languages, including esp. Irish, Scots gaelic, Welsh, and Breton, which survive now in Ireland, the Scottish Highlands, Wales, and Brittany." (http://dictionary.reference.com)

Christianity-"The Christian religion, based upon belief in Jesus as the Christ and upon his teachings" (http://www.yourdictionary.com).

Doctrine of Signatures-"The concept that the key to humanity's use of various plants was indicated by the form of the plant. The red sap of the bloodroot (*Sanguinaria canadensis*), for instance, was believed to cure diseases of the blood, while the fused leaves of boneset (*Eupatorium perfoliatum*) were used to heal broken bones. The concept was employed by the herbalists of the Renaissance, and was accepted until the latter part of the 19th century" (http://education.yahoo.com).

Druid-"A member of a literate and influential class in Celtic society that included priests, soothsayers, judges, poets, etc. in ancient Britain, Ireland, and France" (http://www.yourdictionary.com).

Gaelic-"Of or pertaining to the Gaels, a Celtic race inhabiting the Highlands of Scotland" http://www.wordnik.com/words/Gaelic.

Healer-"A healer is someone who purports to aid recovery from ill health" (http://www.wordiq.com/definition).

Herbalism-" Western herbalism is a form of the healing arts that draws from herbal traditions of Europe and the Americas, and that emphasizes the study and use of European and Native American herbs in the treatment and prevention of illness" (http://medical-dictionary.thefreedictionary.com).

Magic-"The use of means (as charms or spells) believed to have supernatural power over natural forces" (http://www.merriam-webster.com/dictionary/magic).

Medicine wheel-"The Native American medicine wheel was used for healing almost any illness. The Native Americans believe that the basis for most illnesses is spiritual, and focused on treating the source of the problem rather than symptoms. The medicine wheel focuses on balance and how everything is connected. The Native American Medicine wheel consists of four sections with four colors representing certain properties. The colors are Blue, Red, Green and White representing the North, South, East and West, and each section has a different aspect connected with it a certain animals" (http://www.indians.org/articles/native-american-medicine-wheel.html).

Mysticism-"Vague or ill-defined religious or spiritual belief, especially as associated with a belief in the occult" (http://www.oxforddictionaries.com).

Native American medicine-"According to Ken "Bear Hawk" Cohen, "Native American medicine is based on widely held beliefs about healthy living, the repercussions of disease-producing behavior, and the spiritual principles that restore balance." These beliefs are shared by all tribes. However, the methods of diagnosis and treatment vary greatly from tribe to tribe and healer to healer" (http://www.altmd.com/Articles/Native-American-Medicine-Encyclopedia-of-Alternat).

Religion-"A set of beliefs concerning the cause, nature, and purpose of the universe, esp. when considered as the creation of a superhuman agency or agencies, usually involving devotional and ritual observances, and often containing a moral code governing the conduct of human affairs" (http://dictionary. reference.com/browse/religion.

Superstition-"A belief, practice, or rite irrationally maintained by ignorance of the laws of nature or by faith in magic or chance" (http://education.yahoo.com/reference/dictionary).

Voodoo-"A religion practiced chiefly in Caribbean countries, especially Haiti, syncretized from Roman Catholic ritual elements and the animism and magic of slaves from West Africa, in which a supreme God rules a large pantheon of local and tutelary deities, deified ancestors, and saints, who communicate with believers in dreams, trances, and ritual possessions" (http:// www.thefreedictionary.com/voodoo).

Witchcraft-"*a*: the use of sorcery or magic *b*: communication with the devil or with a familiar 2: an irresistible influence or fascination" (http://www.merriam-webster.com/dictionary/witchcraft).

Linkage to Traditional Naturopathy

Herbalism has been used throughout history. Naturopathy, as a holistic approach to healing, has herbalism as one of its tenets.

"Naturopathy is a philosophy which encompasses a view of life, a model for living a full life. The word naturopathy is a Latin-Greek hybrid which can be defined as 'being close to or benefiting from nature" (Classical Traditional Naturopathy Information on the Art and Science of Natural Health and Wellness, 2011, p.2)

"The roots of naturopathy are found in the ancient Greece of Hippocrates, who recognized and wrote about the healing power of nature. As a specific discipline, naturopathy is related to the European nature cure, which evolved during the 19th Century. Begun as a result of observing the healing effects of nature, these methods use fresh air, sunlight, water, diet, exercise, and rest to promote health.

Benedict Lust, a German immigrant who is recognized as the father of American naturopathy, first came to the United States in 1892 at age 20. Lust (pronounced "Loost") initiated a movement that he later named naturopathy, which he described as "first instruction, then inspiration, and ultimately growth." From the beginning, naturopathy has been deeply concerned with lifestyle.

The basic tenet of naturopathy is that human life is governed by the same self-regulating, self-repairing forces that care for all living things. Its methods are natural in that they utilize readily available resources such as food and water, but do not require specific products. The traditional naturopath, or naturopathic consultant, can assist clients with identifying the improvements in daily lifestyle that would support the body in self-healing" (Clayton College of Natural Health, 2010, para. 1).

The American Association of Naturopathic Physicians defines Naturopathic Medicine as "a distinct system of primary health care—an art, science, philosophy and practice of diagnosis, treatment and prevention of illness. Naturopathic medicine is distinguished by the principles which underlie and determine its practice. These principles are based upon the objective observation of the nature of health and disease, and are continually reexamined in the light of scientific advances. Methods used are consistent with these principles and are chosen upon the basis of patient individuality. Naturopathic physicians are primary health care practitioners, whose diverse techniques include modern and traditional, scientific and empirical methods" (The American Association of Naturopathic Physicians, 2010, para. 1).

CHAPTER TWO

Introduction of Related Literature and Research

The Native American medicine wheel has been used for centuries as a means of defining the different stages of life. As depicted, it is a circle, as in the circle of life with a cross in the middle (also used by St. Patrick in his conversion of Celtic pagans to Christianity).

In the Native American Indian culture, the cross actually points to the four directions and those directions signify specific states of the human being; spiritual at the north, emotional to the east, physical in the south, and intellectual in the west. Please note that instead of moving in what is termed a Eurocentric pattern and also the direction one uses in making the sign of the cross (north, south, east, west). Indians follow the direction of the sun. The direction of this study will be in using the medicine wheel to break down each of the components presented.

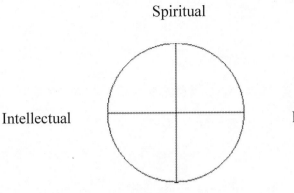

Spiritual

Intellectual

Emotional

Physical

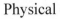

Native American Medicine Wheel-B

Figure 2.

Spiritual

Bonwick (1894) described druids as being "spiritualistic conjurers, dealers with bad spirits, and always opposing the Gospel." He also depicted their role in time as being "evil spirits" and equated them as magicians.

The ancient Celtic society was entrenched in myth, magic, and medicine. Klemens (2008) describes in great detail the impact that druids (shamans and shamankas) had, especially in herbal/natural medicine, as well as in the healing arts and magic. In speaking about druid magic, he describes their use of the four natural elements and corresponding compass points and colors (closely related to the Native American medicine wheel).

Winston (1992) describes Cherokee medicine as being a "system of medical/spiritual knowledge and practices that developed over the last 3,000-4,000 years." In his article, he discusses herbal medicine; physical medicine; dreamwork; language/myths/laws; ceremonies; and the laws of nature. Additionally, he discusses the medicine priest's knowledge and the holistic perspective held by the Cherokee people.

Barish (2010) wrote about Appalachian healthcare in remote communities. He wrote about the unique features of such communities. Among those were "faith healing, including prayer, and family-taught remedies being the most commonly used complimentary and alternative medicine modalities."

Coyne, Damien-Popescu, and Friend (2006) accomplished a study on social and cultural factors in southern West Virginia. Among those factors studied were health care related to faith. One of the findings reported was that there is a distrust of specialists and prescription medicines. Another was that they seek divine help when in need of healing.

Emotional

Researchers studied traditional, complimentary, and alternative medicine among Hispanic and American Indian communities. There were a number of findings regarding perceptions between patients and clinicians. An important one to note is that discussions were avoided out of fear of how the clinician would respond to the patient using herbs as opposed to prescribed medications. Another was that of allopaths criticizing cultural practices such as sweat lodge use (Shelley, Sussman, Williams, Segal, Crabtree, et. al, 2009).

Davies' (1999) research describes the differences between quacks and the cunning-folk and describes the role of herbalism at that point in time. He also shows the role that magic and sorcery played and how they were used in connection with herbalism.

An article written about death brought on through a curse or sorcery discussed the role that fear can play in an individual's death; patients from another culture and becoming ill from a curse or in our culture, from a physician or pathologist who gives a death sentence diagnosis. Additionally, the author discusses that the medical community might accomplish more if it were better versed in traditional healer ways, as well as to add an anthropologist to a social cardiac team when faced with screening individuals for potential cardiac arrest and coronary disease that could present as psychogenic "sudden adult death" (Comfort, 1981, p. 333).

Physical

Lee (2006) connects the history of drugs of antiquity to witches, and then to a homeopathic doctor (Crippen), who was accused of murder. All made use of the herb, henbane. The article describes it as both poison and a narcotic and depicts its use by "witches, wizards, and soothsayers as a compound of their hallucinatory and flying ointments" (para. 1).

The American Red Cross (1996, p. 27) provides insight into the American Indian's holistic approach to health. Stated is that sickness is an imbalance which occurs between a person and his/her universe. Described is the role of traditional healing practiced in the Native culture(s) and the realization that because "the body and soul are one, that health is synonymous with the harmony of body and soul with nature."

Kattleman, Conti, and Ren (2009) studied obesity and diabetes in the Cheyenne River Sioux tribe. They designed a Medicine Wheel Model for Nutrition program in collaboration with tribal leaders and members and performed the program after summer celebrations and before the Christmas holiday in order to ensure participation and success.

An investigation of Navajo practices studied seriously ill Navajos and their use of both traditional and non-traditional modalities of health care. It was found that when traditional Navajo ceremonies are incorporated into Western medicine, more healing is accomplished. The suggestion is made that each of the medicine wheel components must be attended to, in order for harmony of the body to be put into balance (Coulehan, 1980).

According to Webb (1981), a study constructed with both nurses and patients in the New Orleans area defined how voodoo has affected the health of those who believe in it. Next, the author describes some of the techniques, inclusive of herbs used to make the curses, gris-gris bags, charms, amulets, and magical powders used in the rituals and/or for protection or harm.

Intellectual

There are three (3) divisions of druids and their particular roles. The Ovates were the shamans and diviners. The Bards were the musicians and story-tellers. The third and most prominent position was the Celtic Druid who controlled law and judgments, inclusive of executions. Working together, all three struck much fear and awe into the average person, as well as in royalty (History of the Celtic Druids, 2011, para. 2).

Ancient Celtic physicians were touted to be venerated and had extra protections that were afforded them. Ancient laws were very strictly enforced, when what was termed as "quackery" appeared. Additionally, Celtic physicians appreciated the value of cleanliness, pure water, and free ventilation in the treatment of the sick and wounded" ("Ancient Celtic Physicians," 1897).

Blake (2008) deals with the evolution of Native American herbalism, eclectic physicians, and Thompsonian Herbalism. A short history of Samuel Thompson's work is given, therefore giving the reader the stepping-stones to much of modern-day's herbalism.

Emotional

Kwok (1998) conducted a study to determine how much, if any, Navajo native healers were utilized, and/or when used, conflicted with conventional medicine. Two interesting findings were that 1) the native healers were correlated with the Pentecostal faith, and 2) that patients rarely saw conflict between their healers and allopaths.

Research showed that the role of traditional health care providers serving the Appalachian client-base and the subsequent need to look at the role that folk medicine plays in healing. It was found that much of that role is downplayed (Folk Medicine and Health Beliefs: An Appalachian Perspective, 1996).

Struthers, Eschiti and Patchell (2008) identified the need for nurses to integrate traditional indigenous healing into holistic care. They interviewed four Anishiabe medicine men and identified seven themes: "1) The Healing Path, 2) Health as Wholeness, 3) Healing Ways, 4) Healing Stories, 5) Culture Interwoven with Healing, 6) Healing Exchange, and 7) Connection with Western Medicine." The conclusion included health care providers needing to be more knowledgeable in each of the component areas in order to illicit better communication.

Hemphill (1966, p. 901) compared the history of witchcraft and psychiatric illness in Western Europe beginning with the Inquisition and bringing that into modern-day occurrences. Discussed were many of the aspects of witchcraft, including ointments and potions made and the delierient drugs and poisons made from leaves and herbs to induce altered states, then and some discussion about present-day hallucinogens used such as mescaline. Lastly, the author states that "The Church, in the name of Christ, with His message of compassion, tolerance and humility, promotes the witch trials."

Summary

The thrust of this historical perspective and the literature presented will be to give you, the reader, a basic understanding of the past-to-present timeframe, the role of magic, religion, and mysticism, and the subsequent impact and influence that they have had through the ages. Given that history, it is hoped that you will be able to articulate why modern-day herbalism has struggled in some instances, and in other instances, has become a successful means of healing.

CHAPTER THREE

Celtic and Druidic History

The early Celtic nations were Alba (Scotland); Breizh (Brittainy); Cymru (Wales); Eire (Ireland); Kenrow (Cornwall); and Mannin (Man/Isle of Mann). Early Celts, particularly in Ireland, were incredible conservationists. Their primary occupations were in the fields of agriculture and as tradespeople. Their focus on conservation through agriculture was in farming, but also on clearing the woodlands for farming and to build roadways for transportation. Additionally, the dependence on farming included obtaining building materials, dye materials, food for themselves and their livestock, and for healing remedies. They were very reverent of wood that was already cleared, as well as that which was still standing. In fact, there were severe penalties for those who damaged existing trees.

In Ireland, trees and shrubs were equated with social classes. They were divided into "nobles, commoners, lower divisions, or bushes" (Clancy, n.d, p. 3). As each category of tree or shrub was valued, so was each social class for its particular gifts/uses.

Early Celtic society was communal and tribal and centered around faith, their many deities, and nature. Faith was polytheistic, with as many as four hundred (400) deities being worshipped and dependent upon direction of all aspects in their lives by druids.

This included their history, music, poetry, art, and lore being developed and passed on by the Bards. History, with the exception of the Welsh, was oral. Welsh druids were the only early-known druidic society who committed their history/works to paper.

The highest level of druidic society were actually identified as druidic priests. They were the lawyers, judges, astronomers, royal advisors, philosophers, mathematicians, and scholars. In order to reach this level, they were required to apprentice for at least twenty (20) years.

Druids were highly revered, as well as highly feared. The druids in Ireland were actually responsible for the development of Brehon Law. They were considered to be as powerful, and in many cases, more powerful than the royalty they "served." Druids decided all matters of life and death in their communities.

Manner of punishment could indeed be another reason to fear these pillars of the community. It could be meted out in something as trivial as community service or giving back to the "church." However, they were also well-known for very cruel deaths for their own, but especially for captured enemies. One of the most popular methods of death was to put the offender (many times, multiple offenders) into wooden cages and then to burn them alive.

This is just one of the events that the second level of druid, the Ovate, was called upon for their knowledge/craft. The ovate was the one who foretold the future and so, extracted the punishments. The only seeming grace of such a cruel death was that the Ovate (shaman) would drug the prisoner(s), using a mixture of plants and herbs, such as narcotics and hallucinogens, so that they were numb by the time death arrived.

The druidic faith was one centering around nature. They learned all there was to know about nature, herbalism, healing, the history of trees, and what time truly means; why and how it relates to birth, death, and reincarnation. Druids believed in the cycle of life and even had a medicine wheel which closely resembles the Native American Medicine Wheel of today.

NORTH-WEST:
Karma, lessons to be learned, recognizing attachments (events from the past being projected into the future), hopes and fears which we project. Patterns of illusion . . .

NORTH:
Darkness. Midnight. Earth, mountains, landscape, stones and minerals. The Earth Goddess and Horned God. The silver wheel of Arianhrod representing the wheel of stars. Place of ice, frozen potential energy, waiting be born.

NORTH-EAST:
Design of energy, male/female balance, the Sacred Marriage

WEST:
Sunset, dusk, green growing abundance, fecundity and harvesting, the point of change, of death and dying across the waters of the western sea. This is the primary gateway to the underworld, Annwn, the realms beyond physical life.

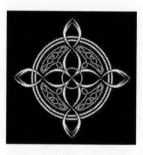

EAST:
Air, sunrise, dawn, place of ideas, new concepts, rebirth, illumination.

SOUTH-WEST:
The dream-weave, the place where the future is being woven, access point to the Web of Wyrd, the tapestry of life . . .

SOUTH:
Fire, midday sun, strongest sun place of energy, expansion and play.

SOUTH EAST:
Ancestors of land and place and personal ancestral memory.

Celtic Medicine Wheel of the British Isles

Figure 3.

(The Celtic Medicine Wheel, p.1)

The oak and mistletoe were/are sacred to druidism, so sacrifices and feasts were both held in oak groves. Both oak and mistletoe were used medicinally and in rituals. Magic, mysticism, potions, and healing arts were used in both feasts and sacrifices.

Feasts centered around astronomy and the changes of season. In fact, the Celtic calendar was developed around these, as well.

Because Ovates were the soothsayers, it was said that they were able to open the doors of time. Ergo, they were seen as the link to reincarnation as they dealt with birth, death, and re-birth.

Tree-lore, herbalism, and healing were the primary areas of study for the Ovates. "The plant world is a great teacher of the laws of death and re-birth, of sacrifice and transmutation and the tree is the supreme teacher of the mysteries of time, with its leaves likewise mostly hidden from us in the heights of the subconscious, holding the potential of the future in the seeds that will in due time fall.

The art of healing concerns the application of natural law to the human body and psyche. If the heart, mind, or body is out of time with nature, we suffer. The application of natural remedies with plants, with the four elements, with solar, lunar, and stellar power were studied by the Ovate" (What Is An Ovate?, 2011, para. 14).

CHAPTER FOUR

Witchcraft

"Sorcery is an attempt to control nature and to produce good or evil results, generally by the aid of evil spirits" (Hemphill, 1966, p. 891). In the medieval era, Christians truly believed that both good and bad spirits could shape-shift. They also believed that Satan had been empowered by God to set things in motion on earth and to work toward possessing souls.

Witchcraft has permeated all stratas of society. History has shown the damage it has wrought in the areas of "science, medicine, culture, and humanity" (Robbins, 1959; Hemphill, 1966, p. 891).

The Inquisition occurred during the twelfth and thirteenth centuries. At that time, the Church declared that the individuals involved were heretics and that through their acts, would be leading others away from said Church. Because of this, the Church sought to get confessions from the accused through torture. If they confessed, they were strangled, then burned. If not, they had to forego being strangled first, but were burned publicly while still alive.

This was then followed by the Reformation and this mentality carried on through the 1800's in Europe, the worst of it being in Scotland, Ireland, and England. There were at least 4400 deaths by fire in Scotland and countless numbers were drowned. The verification process was that if one was a witch, he/she would float while having thumbs and toes bound together; if not, they immediately sank and drowned. Due to this process, thousands were drowned.

At the turn of the twentieth century, the water refuse viaduct in Edinburgh became clogged. When workers went in to clean it, they found countless skeletons and clothing from the victims. It is now known that floating was typically caused by air trapped in women's skirts and those who immediately sank, drowned because their clothes and shoes had become quickly saturated and heavy.

Witches were considered to be both male and female Christians who, as new disciples of Satan, had been imbued with magical powers. The Church later came up with the concept picture of the witch being an old hag as they thought that using one of a young beauty would be too tempting for those who would be swayed.

Witch ceremonies were conducted on what was termed the sabbat. This was where the idea that witches rode on brooms came from (originally it was "rakes"). In these ceremonies, they worshipped Satan and performed all manner of perverse acts. In

Scotland, the sabbat was said to be akin to "sexual highland games at which whisky was distributed" (Hemphill, 1966, p. 894).

Flying ointment was used by witches to fly or to shape-shift. Some witches sold killing ointments/powders, potions, and charms which could be used for harm or for sexual purposes. Henbane was popular with witches, wizards, and soothsayers in flying ointments due to its hallucinogenic properties (Lee, 2006, para. 1).

Witches were purported to have caused death through epidemics by being "plague-smearers." They were reported to have made smearing ointments from corpses and then to have put them on houses.

Ancient witches were often guised as healers. They were often known as cunning-folk and charmers and were a part of what was known as the medical "black-market" (Davies, 1999, p. 56). Many were considered to be "high-street herbalists or irregular practitioners," but had other occupations which were typically not connected to the medical field.

Unfortunately, many were branded as quacks and were condemned for promoting "superstitious credulity." Cunning-folk, however, were those who said that they had magical powers. Quacks tended to move around, as opposed to the cunning-folk who typically stayed close to home. Quacks, because of their nomadic lifestyle had to advertise (hence, the nickname "quack," as in the honking sound a duck makes), whereas cunning-folk did not.

Both the cunning-folk and quacks practiced urine-scrying. Quacks advertised their medicines as being cure-alls and for specific diseases, but didn't typically practice astrology or magic. However, cunning-folk were usually sought out to work with persistent illnesses that the allopathic physicians couldn't treat; strange fits of depression, and others such as lice-infestation were considered to be bewitchment.

When witchcraft was suspected, people generally had two (2) alternatives; private counter-magic or meeting with a cunning-person. Orthodox doctors and chemists typically had some working knowledge of the occult, but rarely had what they considered to be the power to counter witchcraft.

CHAPTER FIVE

Celtic Women as Healers

The role of ancient Celtic women as healers, priestesses, shamankas, medicine-women, oracles, diviners, and/or wise-women has been one of both empowerment and disempowerment through subordination, as has been seen historically for women, in general, through history. This has been attributed to power struggles, many times involving the Church, and done to undermine female power, subordinating them to men, as in the Christian dogma (women subordinate to men, as man is to the church, as the church is to Christ). In fact, the Bible disempowers women with the dictates that women are to be kept are to be separated from men and quiet concerning church matters. Additionally, King James edited the Bible and in his version, had women taken out of leadership roles.

Interesting to note, is that women in priestess, healer, teacher, counseling and leadership roles, have been those who have been open to attack and it is women who are cast into primary roles of evil, such as in witchcraft and the dark arts, while having equal/

lateral skills, but being subordinated by gender in role. What a paradox to Christianity, which puts the female on a pedestal as a maternal figure to be respected, revered, and honored.

Both druids and Christians use the cross as symbols. "Interestingly, the Celtic Cross was enclosed by a circle, for spirit, the turning of the wheel. The Circle is Feminine, to the spokes' angular Masculine. The Christian Cross elongated to the Masculine and shrank the Feminine until it was usually gone completely" (Druidry & Christianity, 2011, para. 4).

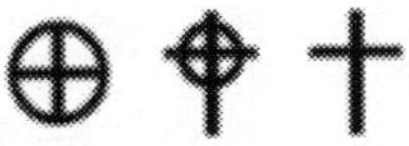

⊕ ⊕ ✝

Celtic and Christian Crosses

Figure 4.

Throughout history, this is seen multiple times. For example, Joan d'Arc was charged with witchcraft, which "arose in her initial contact with the aristocracy, years before her Inquisitorial trial, and her stance of prophetic power and divine inspiration played a role in her execution" (priestesses, power, and politics).

In 60 A.D., Boadicea, married to King Prasutagus of the Icenian nation, became a widow. Her husband, during his reign, had assured, through his will, that upon his death, his wife and two teen-aged daughters, would inherit his wealth and the small Briton kingdom. At this time, Iceni was an independent ally of Rome. However, upon his death, the Roman governor, Paulinus decided otherwise.

It was his belief that, as he desired Iceni for his own, that he didn't have to follow Briton law. He marched troops into Iceni, pillaged their castles, flogged Boadicea unmercifully for standing up to them and then made her watch as her two children were brutally raped. Roman women would have cowered and become submissive, but not so in a Celtic woman, and queen at that. Once recovered, she vowed vengeance and revenge, not only for herself, but for her daughters, her deceased husband, and his kingdom.

A fierce figure she was to behold; she rode by chariot with her daughters by her side from village to village, rallying country men and women to stand against the Romans; a feat heretofore unheard of, especially by a woman, which of course, led to monumental humiliation for the Romans, a male-dominated culture.

She led her troops, made up of men and women, boys and girls, through Roman town after town, totally decimating everything in their path. No Roman man, woman, child, or home was left. It is estimated that they killed over 70,000.

Her final battle saw Druids lined up shouting curses to the heavens and black-cloaked women with hair flying and holding torches high, screaming like banshees. The Roman soldiers had never lay witness to battle such as this and were scared into an eerie quiet. Boadicea rode her chariot into the fray, leading some 230,000 into battle.

The fight was fast and furious. She lost close to 80,000 as the Romans used shields and short swords to push back and slay the once-mighty Britons. It was as if a wall of metal had been formed and kept pushing them back. The battle became a massacre of the Britons, as only 400 Romans were lost. It is recounted that when the queen saw what had been lost, she took her own life with deadly nightshade (Matthews, 1988 & Wilde, 1997, p. 2).

Even writers such as "Joyce (writing in the early 20th century) added almost as a footnote: It is worthy of remark that in our legendary history, female physicians are often mentioned: and so we see that in ancient Ireland the idea was absurd which is so extensively coming into practice in our own day." Thompson (2010, para. 3) attributes that change of role for women to the Roman church.

CHAPTER SIX

Voodoo

Voodoo in Louisiana, as well as having spread north with the Hurricane Katrina migration, is still very much alive in the United States. The roots of voodoo originate from Africa and with the slave trade, having moved with slaves to Haiti and then primarily into the New Orleans area. It stemmed as a spiritual practice/religion for slaves and became coupled with Catholic practices forced onto them by their "owners." Voodoo, coupled with Catholicism is polytheistic in that though they believe in one God as the Creator, they still pray to and worship minor deities and spirits for everyday activities. It is kept alive more through oral tradition than by wrote materials, such as the Christian Bible (Voodoo Queens, 2010, p. 1).

Components of what is known as New Orleans voodoo include these deities/spirits for "help, advice, and support through prayer, divination, and magic. Herbalism also plays a major role in New Orleans voodoo, where it is known as Hoodoo, or root doctoring, and the voodoo priest and priestess are often powerful healers, working with herbs and with more spiritual and magical healing tools" (The Llewelyn Encyclopedia: Term Voodoo, 2010, para 1).

It came to the US in the 1700's. Because Louisiana and New Orleans, in particular, was a new area and a small number of plantationists owned large numbers of slaves each, the African culture was allowed to continue to exist. In addition to that, the Embargo Act of 1808 stopped slave trade and in so doing, promoted families to be raised and sold together, stopping separation of family members. Because of this lack of separation and the high mortality rate of slaves, the culture and language which was brought over, stayed within the families and the slave communities, bringing them ever closer together.

Louisiana voodoo incorporates the use of spirits (lou), which are used in everyday matters such as life, love, family, and justice. "In voodoo, there are many loua. Although there is considerable variation among families and regions, there are generally two groups of loua, the rada and the petro. The rada spirits are mostly seen as "sweet" loua, while the petro are seen as "bitter" because they are more demanding of their "children." Rada spirits appear to be of African origin while petro spirits appear to be of Haitian origin" (Haitian Voodoo, 2010, para. 4).

These spirit deities originally had African names, but once in Louisiana, began to take on the names of Catholic saints. New Orleans voodoo also uses other components of the Catholic faith, such as the Hail Mary, using the sign of the cross, the Lord's Prayer, and baptism. Coincidentally, the spirits and saints were/are mediators to Mother Mary and Legba (spirit-god), much as a Catholic priest is the intercessor to Christ. Additionally, Legba is equated with St. Peter as they are both considered to be the "guardians of the gates."

In the 1800's, the role of voodoo priests became replaced in primary power by priestesses. In the early 1830's, this role became the strongest in US history, as Marie Laveau began her reign as the voodoo queen. Known as "Mamzelle," she acted as an oracle/diviner and also performed exorcisms and made sacrifices to the spirits. She was a devout Catholic, adopting even more of the religion into her voodoo practices. Laveau was the eighth generation of African-Haitian voodists. Both parents practiced the black arts and all women in her lineage were specialists in the voodoo religion. In addition to other Catholic symbols already being used, Marie added the use of holy water, incense, and statues to rituals. Additionally, she promoted Catholicism to her followers.

Marie Laveau was a hairdresser by trade and used the secrets she heard as idle gossip in the salon to blackmail many. She had a network of spies who both loved and feared her, gathering information and being paid in-kind with free sessions with the queen. These included both healing spells and curses. Additionally, Mamzelle used powerful gris gris (charms) and brute force to control others. She was known for having incorporated orgies, using local black, mulatto, and quadroon women to pleasure white men. She opened her rituals and ceremonies up to the public, the press, to police, and to thrill-seekers.

Ceremonies and ritualistic dances were always conducted by the priestesses. In private, they were able to earn an income through the making and provision of gris-gris, charms, potions, powders, and amulets used to cure ills, to confuse or destroy others, and/or to grant desires.

Impressions that lay-people have of voodoo involves both the use of voodoo dolls and of turning the dead into zombies. Voodoo dolls are a form of gris gris and associated with sympathetic magic. They were originally used to bless, not to curse, as commercialization has led society to believe. Where a pin is said to be stuck into the doll to cause pain, the original ones were used for love, prosperity, power, and/or uncrossing (removing a curse). This was done by pinning either a name or a picture of a person onto the doll.

Zombies were glamorized by Hollywood as being deceased individuals raised back to life after having been buried. Zombies were to have no will and were supposedly under another's control. In reality, zombies are live people, who are under the influence of powerful, mind-altering drugs. These drugs are said to be administered by what are known as evil sorcerers. This is done more in Haiti than in the United States (Vodun (a.k.a. Voodoo and related religions, 2010, para. 7).

Snakes/serpents play an important role for the priestess in dances and ceremony in New Orleans voodoo. The snake is used as a prophet. Two (2) interesting points here are that the snake is used in Appalachian magic and in some churches for the same purpose and the snake is also associated with St. Patrick, who was reputed to have driven all of the snakes out of Ireland (Christian myth or magic?).

Louisiana voodoo rituals appear to be quite eclectic, taking bits and pieces from other religions and spiritual practices, such as African Yoruba, Catholicism, Satanism, and even the Native American culture. Rituals are typically held in a temple with a middle pole, which is where God and spirits can communicate with individuals. There is an altar present which is decorated with symbols such as candles, pictures of saints, etc.

Rituals begin with a feasting. A veve (flour or cornmeal circle) is placed on the floor. Ceremony is held within that circle. A rattle and drum(s) are used and chanting begins. The priest(ess) and any apprentices dance. Dancing becomes more intense as the dancer's spirit leaves his/her body and another spirit possesses his/her body. Whoever the dancer is, is treated with ultimate respect by all present.

Animal sacrifices (equated with Abraham and the lamb) are conducted. When the neck of the animal is slit, the blood is collected. Once collected, the dancer may drink of it. By sacrificing in this manner, it is said that the spirits' hunger is appeased. The animal is then typically cooked and eaten. This process is equated with Christian communion.

A voodoo spell which was called a cure-all was one that could solve all problems. "The cure-all was a Voodoo spell that could solve all problems. There were different recipes in Voodoo spells for cure-all; one recipe was to mix jimson weed with sulphur and honey. The mixture was placed in a glass, which was rubbed against a black cat, and then the mixture was slowly sipped" (Louisiana Voodoo, 2010, para.22).

Fear is a primary control element of the voodoo priests and priestesses. In *Voodoo Death* (Cannon, 1942), "suggested that voodoo death is the result of shock produced by the sudden release of adrenalin. The victim breathes rapidly, has a fast pulse, and hemoconcentration caused by loss of fluids from the blood to the tissues. The heart beats at an extremely fast rate leading to a state of constant contraction and to death in systole" (Webb, 1971, p. 293). Subliminal suggestions, superstition, and fear all play a part in voodoo magic.

Other fears and superstitions held involved the fear of "needle doctors." Needle doctors were student doctors who supposedly stuck needles into victims' arms after dark and would then practice all sorts of experiments on them. Because of this legend, it was believed that those who were victimized would never be seen from again, as they were supposedly killed and their bodies used for even more experimentation. This fear was fueled by voodooists, as another means of control and to keep individuals away from orthodox practitioners.

CHAPTER SEVEN

Native American

For the purposes of this book, although many tribes will be attended to relevant to Native American medicine, a stronger focus will be seen on the Cherokee tribe, as it is a primary tribe in the southern part of the United States. Additionally, the Cherokee tribe has had a great impact on the history of the Appalachian culture.

"The Indian way is to live in harmony with the earth and with oneself and to walk with spirit, heart, mind, and body in balance as an integrated being." The Indian culture is based on a "connection between spirituality and wellness. Wellness is harmony in all three aspects of one's being. Being unwell is a disharmony of mind, body, and spirit. Wellness consists of:

1. Thoughts;
2. Concepts; and
3. Application

The concept of spirit, body, and mind interacting in humans is basic to the practice of traditional Indian medicine" (Tulsa Area Chapter, 1996, p. 33). "The Cherokee word "tohi"—health—is the same as the word for peace. You're in good health when your body is at peace" (Cherokee medicine, medicine men and medicine ways, 2010, para. 1).

The Indian culture is steeped in tradition and has a very strong social system. Family is very important and is at the center of almost all activities. This makes perfect sense, given that almost all tribes were matriarchal in the beginning; that changing somewhat with Eurocentric influence. Within Indian society, elders are honored and revered, and with this comes the oral histories and traditions being passed from one generation to the next.

Indian medicine involves many people and from these people, both genders are involved. Among those are singers, midwives, plant/herb doctors/herbalists, medicine men and women, wise men and women, spiritual counselors, elders, diagnosticians, and/or shamen (Crockett, 1971, p. 6).

These traditional healers attend to the body, mind, and spirit, as well as to symptoms and physical ailments. There are many diseases however, which were brought by the white man or are considered to be white-man's diseases. Included, but not limited to, these are smallpox, cancer, diabetes, tuberculosis, and HIV/AIDS. There are no traditional medical treatments for them. Traditional Indians, when faced with a chronic or terminal disease, typically wait to get "regular" medical help until the disease is either out-of-control or it's too late to be of any benefit.

Not all tribes share the same philosophies, but there are symbols that are common to most. One of those is the medicine wheel. It has been used for both spiritual and ritual purposes, and for healing purposes. Because the medicine wheel represents a circle and the circle represents balance, the concept of wellness being harmony and balance and utilization of the medicine wheel for healing works splendidly.

The medicine wheel is a cross within a circle. (Coincidentally, it is the same as the symbol that St. Patrick used many years prior to convert Celts to Christianity). There are four (4) points on the circle and each represents one of the four (4) directions. Each direction, depending on the tribe, might be associated with different animals, minerals, colors, or characters (Dudgeon, n.d., p. 3). The American Red Cross HIV/AIDS training program takes the wheel and assigns different points of one's life to it, using it metaphorically, to describe the progression of HIV/AIDS, as does the Hopi tribe. This assignation is related, as well to Erik Erikson's Stages of

Psychosocial Development. The North represents Childhood; East represents Adolescence; South represents Adulthood; and the West represents Elderhood (Tulsa Area Chapter, 1996, p. 46; Medicine Wheel, 2010, para. 23). In James Mooney's History (1900), the cardinal directions and colors for the Cherokee are as follow:

East = red = success; triumph

North = blue = defeat; trouble

West = black = death

South = white = peace; happiness.

The Anishaabe tribe uses the following colors in their medicine wheel:

COLOR/ DIRECTION	DESCRIPTOR	SEASON	EMOTE	ELEMENT
Blue North	defeat; trouble	winter; a season for survival and waiting	wisdom; intellect; the adult self; MIND	wind/ breath
Yellow East	success; triumph	spring; a re-awakening; the power of new life;	Illumination; creation; the wonder; child self; SPIRIT	fire/life source
Black West	death	autumn; the final harvest; the end of life's cycle	introspection and intuition; the physical body; MANIFESTATION	earth
White South	peace; happiness	summer; a time of plenty	trust and innocence; EMOTIONS	water
Center	learning	balance	beauty; harmony; SELF	

Anishabe Tribal Medicine Wheel Defined

Table 1.

(Native American Medicine Wheels History

and Meaning, para. 7-11)

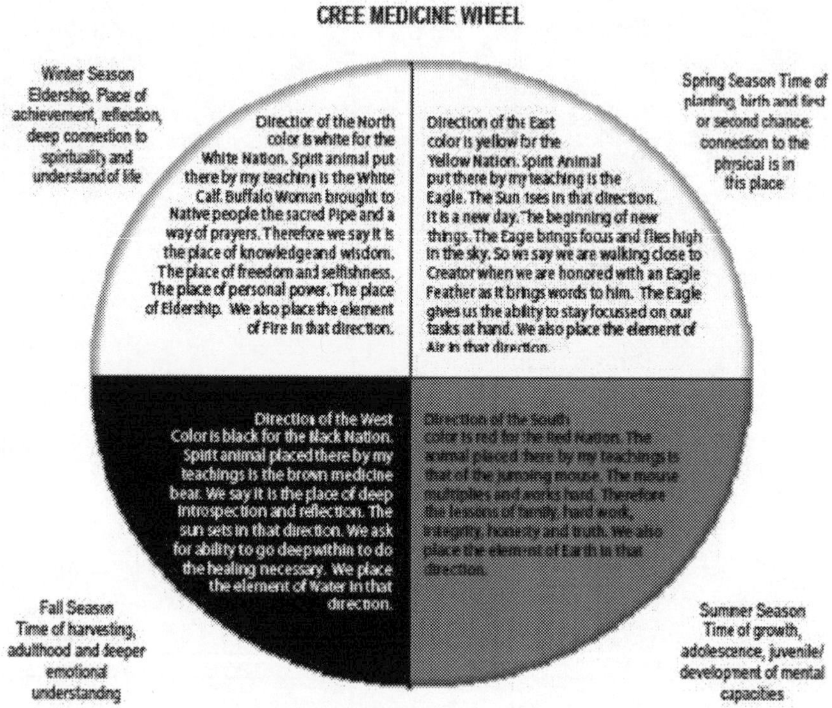

CREE MEDICINE WHEEL

Winter Season
Eldership. Place of
achievement, reflection,
deep connection to
spirituality and
understand of life

Direction of the North color is white for the White Nation. Spirit animal put there by my teaching is the White Calf. Buffalo Woman brought to Native people the sacred Pipe and a way of prayers. Therefore we say it is the place of knowledge and wisdom. The place of freedom and selfishness. The place of personal power. The place of Eldership. We also place the element of Fire in that direction.

Direction of the East color is yellow for the Yellow Nation. Spirit Animal put there by my teaching is the Eagle. The Sun rises in that direction. It is a new day. The beginning of new things. The Eagle brings focus and flies high in the sky. So we say we are walking close to Creator when we are honored with an Eagle Feather as it brings words to him. The Eagle gives us the ability to stay focussed on our tasks at hand. We also place the element of Air in that direction.

Spring Season Time of
planting, birth and first
or second chance.
connection to the
physical is in
this place

Direction of the West Color is black for the Black Nation. Spirit animal placed there by my teachings is the brown medicine bear. We say it is the place of deep introspection and reflection. The sun sets in that direction. We ask for ability to go deep within to do the healing necessary. We place the element of Water in that direction.

Direction of the South color is red for the Red Nation. The animal placed here by my teachings is that of the jumping mouse. The mouse multiplies and works hard. Therefore the lessons of family, hard work, integrity, honesty and truth. We also place the element of Earth in that direction.

Fall Season
Time of harvesting,
adulthood and deeper
emotional
understanding

Summer Season
Time of growth,
adolescence, juvenile/
development of mental
capacities

Directions and Their Meanings

Figure 5.

(The Medicine Wheel, p. 3)

As the reader will note by the figures presented, different tribes attribute colors, symbols, and metaphors differently, but the same basic concept ensues. Each use the circle and the wheel concept to communicate ideas.

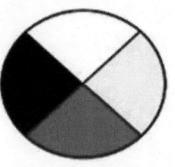

White for North representing preservation

PRESERVATION: BODY - skills - maintaining the positive
patterns and view of life as an on-going system.
Recognizes that Aboriginal people are spirit, heart, mind
and body.

Black for West building on your
life's lesson

BUILDING: DEVELOPING THE
MIND - gaining knowledge,
developing the new positive
life experiences into
continuous patterns and
change the view of life which
includes integrating the
strengths already acquired by
the

Yellow for East representing
awareness

AWARENESS: ATTITUDES AND
INSIGHTS into behavioural
patterns, ever-increasing
understanding of one's self and
the world.

Red for South where you pray for your struggles

STRUGGLE: HEART - feelings about self and others and
how we interrelate - efforts and attempts to change
negative life experiences to positive feeling and believing
that my behaviours influence all of my relations.

A Medicine Wheel of Life's Learning

Figure 6.

(The Medicine Wheel, p. 3)

Circles are very important within the culture. There is the sacred hoop, which was the original medicine wheel. They "were constructed by laying stones in a particular pattern on the ground. Most medicine wheels follow the basic pattern of having a center of stone(s), and surrounding that is an outer ring of stones with "spokes" or lines of rocks radiating from the center." They are used by Indians for "astronomical, ritual, healing, and teaching purposes" (Medicine Wheel, 2010, para. 2). Circles are indicative of nature and the circle of life, which has no beginning and has no end. Circles were used in many ways. An example would be when the Lakota Sioux planned their communities, as all tipis were placed in a circle.

As previously mentioned, the matriarchal role of many tribes has changed. For some, this means that only males are in the medicine person's role. The Cherokee tribe, however, has both medicine men and women. Cherokee "medicine people are taught by other medicine people, who hand down this 'medicine' to the chosen ones. Medicine formulas, songs, and other rites are hand-written in ledgers which have been handed down throughout many years. It is dangerous to try to interpret them without the proper training, as most are written in cryptic fashion, leaving out major portions that the practitioner has learned verbally, written in code, or even written backwards" (Cherokee Medicine Men and Women—Cherokee Nation, 2010, para. 1). Cherokee medicine is called "nevwoti". It is knowledge, skills, and practice which has been developed over the last 3-4,000 years.

The Cherokee and most other Southwestern tribes believe that there are two (2) kinds of medicine people; good and evil. Because the Cherokee also believe in witchcraft (ordinary and killer witches), when a medicine cure doesn't work, it is believed that witchcraft is at work through an evil medicine person and that is deemed to be bad medicine.

These medicine people apprentice for fifteen to twenty (15-20) years. Part of the knowledge that they must gain is that of 400-600 plants. They learn how to use them in ritual and ceremony, in healing, and learn all about the plant signatures.

They are also considered to be conjurers. They learn how to "enlist the aid of spirits and elemental powers to change things, to heal or doctor, to change one's mind, to bring luck, and to protect the sick or weak from negative influences. In some Christian churches, this is called faith healing" (Crockett, 1971, p. 405).

Cherokee (as well as other tribes) healers and traditionalists are gifted with the skills of gathering, use, and preparation of medicinal herbs. These are used in ritual and ceremony, and in healing. Indian medicine people, as previously mentioned, treat the mind in addition to the body. Medicine bundles, which are equated with charms, are used. Herbs and other objects/substances, such as tobacco, bones, feathers, stones, hair, and beads might be used in the "medicine." Medicine bundles are used for "healing, love, business, and sorcery" (Crockett, 1971, p. 405.).

Some tribes consider a medicine person to also be an herbalist. This is true of the Cherokee who hold this person in the highest esteem, but the Navajo consider the herbalist to be the "lowest and most insignificant of the Navajo practitioners" (Crockett, 1971, p. 405).

"Like cures like" is a very important part of Indian medicine. "Yellow plants are good for jaundice; red ones are good for the blood. Some part of the plant might resemble the organ of the body it is designed to cure. The form and the Indian name for ginseng indicated its value to the Penobscots for worms, snakeroot for fits or contortions are determined by their appearance" (Methods of Treatment, 2010, p. 2).

Lockhart (1983, pp. 8-14) lists many plant and herbal healings used by Indians:

- Willow soup was used for pain and bleeding as were the puffball mushroom and bloodroot.
- Sweet fern leaves were used for poison ivy.
- Devil's club tea was used for the control of diabetes and has been said to cure cancer.
- Corn stalk juice was used to clean wounds.
- Goldenseal was used by Cherokees as an antibiotic. They also used Calamus for "colds, colic, heartburn, and indigestion."

- Seminoles chewed spirit weed for boldness, while the Cheyenne chewed Anaphalis margaritacea for strength and protection when warring.

- Echinacea was used for "blood poisoning, gangrene, infections, rabies, smallpox, and snakebites."

- Herbs were used in rituals and healings, such as Hopi pipe ceremonies. These are used to pray to the Creator and bring back spiritual and physical health, and

- The Plains Indians, including the Dakotas, Omaha, Ponca, and Pawnee use Echinacea and red cedar as a smoke for headaches. Some tribes pour infusions of herbs over coals and inhale the smoke to treat respiratory complaints.

CHAPTER EIGHT

Appalachian Medicine

Healers, witches, witch doctors, water witches, witchcraft, Granny Women, Granny Magic, Appalachian Magic, "the Craft," faery folk" magic, "haints," wand, dowsing rod, herbalism, herb doctors, folk medicine, wildcrafting, snake healing, faith healing, homemade remedies, superstition, religion, tradition, and storytelling; all are terms used to describe different aspects of Appalachian Medicine. Appalachian Medicine is a compilation of different cultures. Eires and Scots (Irish and Scottish) both began to immigrate to the Appalachian Mountain region in the 1700's, in an attempt to escape both religious persecution and to try to forge a better way of life due to the extremely poor economic and living conditions they had experienced in their countries of origin.

With them, they brought many traditions, healing skills, lore, superstitions, and religious beliefs that became entwined with those of the Cherokee (then called Tsalagi) Indians, as well as blacks who had originally come over as slaves and settled in that area. The

Appalachian Mountain region is one which covers "Mississippi to New York and includes eleven states within its official boundaries" (Stone, 2010, p. 1).

Appalachian folk medicine has been passed down orally and primarily through families for hundreds of years. It wasn't until the mid-twentieth century that remedies began to be written. Because of the isolation in Appalachia (due to the mountainous terrain), families have stayed cohesed in traditions and customs, in fact, the whole culture, has stayed immersed in the past. Family is one of the strongest components of the Appalachian culture. When geographical and economic isolation are factored in, it makes sense that families have stayed as tight and dependent upon one another as they have. Much of the medicine, having been passed from one generation to the next, has stayed within the family unit and is based on that particular family's history and traditions, dating back to life in their country-of-origin. This includes storytelling, one's particular style of folk medicine, his/her apprenticeship, or matters concerning day-to-day life.

Much of the behavior and many of the remedies are based on superstitious beliefs. These are blended with herbal tradition and knowledge of what heals the body and the soul. Appalachians are typically very fundamental in their religious practice and beliefs, yet have found a way to incorporate religion into the mix, as well.

Witchcraft is/was a very practical part of the Appalachian culture. However, it's very different from the conventional definition of witchcraft, what those outside of that culture envision it as being. The witchcraft practiced in Appalachia is one which relied upon the gifts of Mother Nature. The belief is in "one universal God (the "Creator," the "Maker"). They do, however, observe the sabbats, solstices, and equinoxes, but do not relate them to mythology; it's the seasonal changes they recognize" (MEDEA Study Guide, 2009, p. 6).

This form of healing and magic became known as Granny Magic and the magic and healing was performed by Granny Women. These healers were an integral part of the culture. "Appalachian Granny Magic wasn't quite a religion, not quite a secular practice. Magic and religion and practical concerns became one path, out of which many skilled midwives and herbalists and lay preachers were created" (MEDEA Study Guide, 2009, p. 4).

Due to minimal or no access to physicians or health care in general, reliance on these practitioners was extensive. Granny Women wore many hats. Among those, they acted as midwives and were called in even when a physician had been called. In the event that a doctor couldn't make it, they were there to deliver. If he did, then the Granny Woman would either assist and/or stay to care for the newborn and the new mother. They didn't charge fees, so if they were the primary "doctor," their concern wasn't that it be a quick delivery, as time wasn't their main concern.

Granny Women used herbal remedies, superstition, and were not opposed to the using pharmaceuticals if and when the need arose. Their training was through years of experience and apprenticeship. At that point in time, the majority of women were illiterate (another reason for oral tradition). However, there were those who could read and those few carried what was called a "Midwife's Book," which was used in the event that they had to attend to a complicated delivery.

In the event that herbal remedies such as blackberry tea (for hemorrhaging), raspberry tea (to relax uterine muscles), slippery elm bark (for speeding up delivery), or willow bark tea (for pain relief) didn't work, the Granny Women had no problem with the use of pharmaceuticals. Local drugstores always had supplies of morphine and quinine available over-the-counter, therefore, if pain were a major issue, a morphine tablet was readily available.

Granny Women and Appalachians in general, were very superstitious. Witch doctors and water witches were very common and held in high esteem within each community. In fact, being known as the "local witch" was considered to be an honor. Each title spoke of specific skills, but it wasn't uncommon for one person to possess the skills of both.

The "witch doctor" was one who practiced midwifery, healing, tended to sick children, and practiced magic. In both "practices," the work was sometimes referred to as conjuring or working.

The "water witch" was she who made charms and potions, worked with water dowsing, energy vortexes, and ley lines. She was more likely to be involved with mill magic than the "witch doctor" (Stilwell, 2001, para. 8).

The Appalachian area is so isolated that many practices and traditions from the countries of origin continued, whereas in areas outside of there, became modernized. With modernization, traditions and culture changed; not so in Appalachia. The unfortunate piece is that, because of oral tradition, original meanings of customs, traditions, wisdom, and spells have changed or gotten lost.

Many of the traditions and customs surround lore such as faeries and the ancestral dead (sometimes referred to as "haints"). The faery lore is brought from Europe, where faeries, leprechauns, brownies, sprites, and magical creatures such as selkies and waterhorses were a common part of the culture.

The Cherokee (Tsalagi) have their own version of the "little people," called Yunuwi Tsusdi (pronounced Yowee Uoodskee), and of course, the slaves still had their spirit deities from Africa. With all four cultures, the lore of the "wee people" remained and evolved to fit the new land and new life.

The Tasalgi believed that the Yunuwi Tsusdi lived in the forest and that they could be a help or a menace. Few could/would see them, but of those that did, what was seen was likened to miniature versions of warriors. In fact, one of the beliefs was that if you had offended one (perhaps by not leaving a food offering), that sharp pain one might feel in his/her calf while walking, could be the result of having been shot with a miniature arrow.

The faerie lore/faith was very similar. "The body of practice that works specifically with Faery and otherworld beings is called Faery Seership" (Foxwood, 2009, p. 4). Faeries are known by many names, including but not limited to: faeries, Them, Little People, Sidewise Folk, and the Gentry.

Those practicing in this area knew more than the average person about faeries and spirits. They knew where these and other spirits lived and how to contact them. Additionally, they knew what to do when they were menacing or how to harness the good.

Similar to the Cherokee, it was known that one should leave food for the little people. In so doing, that individual would stay on their good side and be blessed with luck and good wishes. They were considered to be like family, and as family was central to the culture, one must take care of his/her own. To not do so, would be to bring wrath and fury down on and individual and his/her family and life and luck both could become very ugly.

The ancestral spirits were an important part of the culture and the magic, as well. The spirits of the dead and the little people both lived in the woods, in the mountains, in graveyards, by water sources, and by the crossroads (perhaps where the blues legend re: meeting the devil at the crossroads and trading one's soul for fame or fortune evolved from).

Those working with faery seership worked with these spirits and sometimes termed them as "haints" (what we now call ghosts or poltergeists), Grey Ladies, Grey Men, Devil Dogs, the Woods Folk, and Bogans (what we now call "boogey men or booger monsters).

Events such as death were known more as "visits" or "visitations." These visits heralded the arrival of personages such as "Old Man Death" or "Mr. Death" (what we now sometimes refer to as the "Grim Reaper"). Even God was known as "the Creator" or "the Maker," as opposed to his Biblical name.

The "local witch" had charms, spells, and rituals that were used to keep bad spirits away. In fact, the color blue was one used to repel evil forces. A specific shade of blue was used to dispel these spirits and is still used today. It is called "Haint Blue."

Music was a large part of spells and rituals and included singing, dancing, jigs, reels, lullabies, and chants. Those chants were often sung in rounds. Dancing changed from traditional Irish step dancing to what is now known as clogging. This may have changed due to the fact that shoes were scarce in the Appalachia, so when made weren't as delicate as they were in Ireland, so when made here, were made heavy and durable to match the rugged terrain (Irwin, 1985, chapter 5).

Festivals were seasonal and music, being a part of festival and rituals tradition, and were a part of the Irish, Scottish, and Cherokee cultures. Where the Cherokee had ceremonies such as the Earth Blessing and had particular song and drumming, an example of an Appalachian carryover from Europe, would be the singing of *Auld Lang Syne* from Scotland, and written by Robert Burns. Where we are now familiar with this song being sung on New Year's and at Scottish Gatherings such as Burn's Night, it was sung in the Appalachia on Samhain (known to us as Halloween), during funerals, and for the secular New Year.

Witches used other forms of "magic" and ritual in their practice. Divining was popular and took many forms. One that was handed down from European witchcraft and used by the Cherokee as well, was the reading of spiderwebs. The belief was that there were magical messages spun into the webs and only a chosen few could read and interpret them. In fact, a form of lace making was patterned after this and remains as a cottage-industry in some places.

Other types of readings were accomplished using tea leaves, playing cards, tarot cards, clouds, and through scrying, using dirt, sand, or water. Scrying is basically gazing at something and being able to discern, perceive, interpret, or reveal messages. Modern-day literature and Hollywood have equated this with crystal ball or mirror gazing or reading water in a scrying bowl.

Divining rods were used and those changed to "wands." The wand was a very important tool, used in rituals and spells, to accomplish many tasks such as locating water for wells, finding missing objects or persons, finding or sending energy, locating or connecting to spirits, etc.

Many other items were used in ritual. Among those were pottery, baskets, brooms, and candles, all of which were homemade goods. Mirrors were a luxury and rare, but used and where chalices or goblets were used in Europe, a very accessible and well-used item was used in its place; the cast-iron cauldron.

While the Cherokee used it for cooking and to boil water down to obtain salt to be used in cooking and for ceremony (such as "holy salt"), the Appalachians used them for cooking, making soap and candles, and being utilitarian, were used by local witches in the preparation of remedies, charms, and potions. In point-of-fact, it was not at all uncommon to find one in a witch's yard, designating that she was working.

The local witch usually worked alone. She wasn't known to wear a particular style of dress when performing spells or rituals, as is depicted in the books and movies of today.

There were individuals who only practiced, using charms. They were called "charmers." This was a practice that was documented in Europe, showing up in both Celtic and Manx literature, and brought over and continued in the Appalachia for at least 300 years.

Another interesting practice was the use of prayer water. In Ireland and Scotland, for example, particular wells, springs, and lochs are said to have holy, magical, or mystical power, and exist to this day. A few examples of these would be St. Brigid's Well, Glendaloch, and Islan Munde.

St. Brigid's Well is located in County Kildare, Ireland. It is an area of prayer, where drinking of the well water is touted to lead to both physical and spiritual healing. It also of cloth of some import to the person tying it, his/her wishes or prayers will be granted.

Glendaloch, Ireland was the first monastical community in Ireland and sits besides St. Kevin's Cross and the lake where St. Kevin's cave was. The area is magical and mystical in and of itself, but is also an area where the magical white horses live. Simply being near those waters is touted to be a holy experience.

Islan Munde, an island in the loch outside of Ballychulish, Scotland, is an island where only the chieftains of three clans are buried. The spirit of the last chieftain to be buried inhabits and protects all of those who have passed before, until the next one passes, is buried, and takes over that task. It is these histories and many others, which bring forward the making and using of prayer water.

Prayer water was used for blessing and anointing, and through the use of it, it was believed that God would heal an individual (much like holy water or holy oil in the Church and holy salt in the Indian culture). Water sources, such as wells, springs, and spring-fed lakes have long been revered as being magical and mystical, and even portals to the otherworld.

Snake handling is a practice that has unfortunately been equated with Appalachian medicine, but actually didn't come into practice until the early 1900's and is used only minimally to this day. The practice of snake handling is an offshoot of some of the Pentecostal churches and has been outlawed in most states. There is no herbalism used in the practice. However, because it evolved in the Appalachian region, has been connected with it. Though it was initially practiced in the Appalachians, it has been seen in small churches in places such as Punkin' Holler, Oklahoma (where Timothy McVey stayed prior to the Oklahoma City bombing).

Mark 16:17-18 states, "And these signs shall follow them that believe; in my name shall they cast out devils; they shall speak with new tongues; They shall take up serpents; and if they drink any deadly thing, it shall not hurt them; they shall lay hands on the sick, and they shall recover" (Holy Bible, 1977, p. 597). This is the premise for those involved in the practice of snake handling. Those that practice it are fundamentalists, are typically in rural areas, typically maintained through families as tradition, and have taken that particular scripture as the total truth, professing that if one is in the faith, that being bitten cannot harm them. "According to one explanation . . . serpent handling is an act of faith defined by a biblical text" (Tidball and Toumey, 2007, para 1). This particular denomination emphasizes "an individualistic faith, often characterized by such spiritual practices as evangelism, speaking in tongues, and faith healing" (Snake Handlers, 2010, p. 1).

Faith healers are individuals who lay hands on others who are ill and heal through touch and the speaking of Biblical scripture. The premise is that these individuals are vessels of God and the healing happens through the connection through them and from God. Their healing gifts are in these areas:

1. Burns;
2. Bleeding not related to natural causes; and
3. Thrush.

Some of the healers practice in only one area, some in two, and still others practice in all three areas.

For those who deal with burns, they "blow out" or draw the fire out. They contend that fire is contained within a wound and if it isn't taken out, will burn all the way to the bone.

The second area of illness is bleeding. These healers work with both humans and animals.

The last ailment is "Thrash" or "Thrush." Because blisters around the mouth and the subsequent pain are so bad, some babies cannot nurse. These healers contend that those blisters can go all the way through to the digestive tract and become fatal.

Faith healers use a different Bible verse for every ill that they treat. However, though they are all over the Appalachian area, scripture and not plant medicine is the modality that they treat with (Wigginton & Bennett, 1977, pp. 346-347).

Appalachian medicine has evolved from both European herbalism and Native American plant medicine. Besides Granny Women, both men and women were and are also herbal doctors or herbalists. Many of the same remedies were used and new ones introduced. The overriding theme remained(s) the same throughout the literature re: knowledge, skill, and respect for the use and availability of plants for healing:

"There's a plant for every disease. Of course you need to know when to get your herbs. Now, the Indians wouldn't gather no kind of herb unless it was in full bloom. Said it had more strength then" (Irwin, 1985, p. 135).

"I always did believe that God never did make no mistakes. He never made anything he didn't make a remedy for. The Lord's put something out there if we would only get out there and hunt it" (Patton, 2004, p. 13).

"Everything that grows was put here for a reason and it's our jobs t' find out what it's here for" (Carpenter, Page, & Wigginton, 1983, p. 121).

As was noted previously, even the herbalism practiced today and within the last century, was passed down from generation-to-generation, and typically in families. However, as times have changed and culture has evolved slowly in the Appalachia region, apprentices have been chosen outside of the familial circle because of their interest, love, and respect for the field, as well as their natural-born and innate skills, knowledge, and abilities in herbalism. This is evidenced by individuals such as Darryl Patton, Phyllis Light, and Dr. Lelani Stone Anderson (the Cherokee Medicine Woman).

The *Foxfire* series has taught many remedies and skills, as well as introduced many of those who practiced in the Appalachia. One of the most famous was Aunt Arie. As was typical, she stated, "Mommy taught me lots about the doctoring business. When y' have sickness in th' family and no doctors, you sure learn t' do lotsa ways. You just have to. I can remember all th' doctor business. Yes sir. Cause I lived a long ways from th' doctor. Didn't never get to go t' th' doctor" (Carpenter, Page, & Wigginton, 1983, p. 117).

Alex Stewart (Irwin, 1985, p.135) stated, "Back then, people didn't go off (to a doctor). They went to the woods and got their medicine and made it and they wasn't near as much sickness and disease as they is today. My uncle was a herb doctor and he learnt it mostly to me. He cured diseases that none of the regular doctors could cure. He could cure syphilis when all others failed."

A.L. "Tommie" Bass said that he didn't "claim a cure . . . I just try to give people some ease. Plants used to provide this ease varied greatly. Tommie's immense knowledge of herbal lore encompassed more than 300 plants in his personal pharmacopoeia" (Patton, 2004, p. 11).

Though he made and treated individuals, his knowledge came first from an intense interest in the plants that made up the packaged remedies his family got from local drugstores. Once he began studying the ingredients, he then began to match the plants up and developed his own remedies. In addition to that, Tommie wildcrafted, selling herbs to individuals, herb companies and pharmaceutical companies, consulted in the uses, and taught skills to budding apprentices.

Darryl Patton, MA, ND, Master Herbalist, and Clinical Hypnotherapist, apprenticed under Tommie Bass, even documenting Tommie's life in a book. Darryl has been termed a walking encyclopedia of herbal folklore. In addition to operating his own herbal pharmacy, Darryl teaches as an adjunct professor in the field of mountain medicine and herbalism, advocates in the field, authors and publishes two newsletters (*Stalking the Wild* and *The Southern*

Herbalist), and operates weekend workshops and internship programs which teach herbalism, iridology, and wilderness survival.

Phyllis Light, RH, American Herbalist Guild and former Director of Herbal Studies at Clayton College of Natural Health, is a fourth-generation herbalist and healer. Although she began learning her skills from her Creek/Cherokee grandmother, she also apprenticed under Tommie Bass. In addition to teaching, she has worked in an integrative medical clinic and operates her own herbal consulting business.

Lelanie Stone Anderson is an NGED (Non-Governmentally Enrolled Descendant) Cherokee woman, was an RN, who had been learning about herbology, teaching small workshops here and there, and practicing with those who would accept her assistance. She also wrote columns for a local newspaper once a week.

Since that time, she continues nursing, but has a doctorate in Alternative Medicine and Traditional Naturopathy, is an American Indian Herbalist, and is an author (with eleven books to her credit), columnist, lecturer, teacher, and artist. She is known to many locally as "The Cherokee Medicine Woman."

Lelanie began her journey with herbs as a child, when accompanying her Cherokee grandmother on walks in the Oklahoma countryside. There, she was versed on both herb identification and their uses.

Later, she moved to El Paso, Texas, where she learned more about herbal remedies and mentored under a Pima Indian nurse who led her into a circle of those who would become her guides. Following that, she began using remedies and segued into writing, teaching, research, and other endeavors. That research included/includes both written accounts of ancient herbal remedies and interviewing elders for any verbal herb lore she can glean.

I was privileged to study under her for a short period of time and the statement that she opened with and which she has published many times over and it truly seems to encompass what she teaches was "Indian Medicine is a practical system of thought-it is not merely hocus-pocus and folklore. Individual sources of strength and purpose can be discovered by using the powers of Indian Medicine. These are "Ancient Tools" which have been kept alive throughout the history of man for a significant purpose" (Cherokee Messenger, January 1996, p.1).

When Lelanie begins her classes, she typically qualifies her beliefs about herbal medicine with the following story: As the mother of a newborn baby boy who was refusing to nurse due to thrush, and for whom traditional medicines weren't working, she was at her wit's end and went to stay with her grandmother for the weekend. When she explained the problem, her grandmother went to her workroom, returning with puccoon root and a mortar and pestle. She pounded and ground the root until it became a fine, yellow powder; what many of us know as goldenseal. She then blew it into the infant's mouth a number of times over the next two days. Before the weekend was over, the thrush had been cured.

Like Tommie Bass, Lelanie learned about herbs as she was growing up. Unlike Tommie, she had stepped away from it for a number of years. The incident with her son was what had brought her back.

CHAPTER NINE

Full Circle

Herbalism, mysticism, religion . . . The Celts and druids used nature in every aspect of daily life. Herbalism was used in healing, but also to perpetuate superstition, magic, and the faith. One could be healed or harmed through the use of herbs and plants.

Belladonna (deadly nightshade, as well as the other nightshades), for example, were used both as a pain-reliever and to portend death. It was used as an hallucinogenic and anesthetic for fortune-telling and prophecy, religious rituals, entering otherworlds, and as a poison for murder. The nightshades all contain alkaloids, atropine, and scopolamine.

Mistletoe was used for fertility (in people for barrenness and in ritual, for the prosperity of the land). It was also used as an early cancer agent, and in overdose was used lethally as a poison.

Nettle is another plant used by Celts for both good and evil. Nettle could be used for harm as it stings the skin and affects the eyes, nose, throat, lungs, and/or gastrointestinal tract through the histamine contained therein. On the other hand, it was used to stop bleeding from wounds and in excessive menstruation.

Guelder Rose with its red-to-purple berries was another used for good intent and bad. It's incredibly toxic, so was used as a poison, but also for calming menstrual cramps, stomach cramps, and to relieve hiccups.

St. John's Wort, used in ancient times for melancholy, was also used to ward off dark and evil spirits. It has antiseptic, astringent, and anti-inflammatory qualities, so was used to hasten the healing process.

Last, but not least for the purpose of this research, was comfrey, which was considered to be a staple in most Celtic medicine chests. It grows year-round, so was readily available. It was used for bruising, sprains, and broken bones. Though it should only be used externally, was also used as a poison.

Witch ointments and potions were typically made from the leaves of plants and herbs containing deliriant drugs. Digitalis and belladonna caused the sensation that one was floating or flying. Love potions contained mixtures including, but weren't limited to bones, toads, and prunes. These generally caused sick stomachs and excessive flatulence (most likely not something that would lead to attraction). Arsenic powder was often sprinkled on a victim's clothing over a period of time to bring on death through poisoning.

As mentioned previously, the majority of cunning-folk were competent herbalists. Many of the "medicines" prescribed were considered to be simple tonics. However, there were those who practiced what was known as sympathetic magic. They made cocktails from plants whose properties included toxic, narcotic, and hallucinogenic properties. These were typically known as witches' flying ointments (Lee, 2006, p. 67). Bryony and hemlock were among these. The potions were used to both induce and extend illnesses.

Cunning-folk were known as well, for performing abortions. Among the herbs used for this were feverfew (known also as "kill-bastard"), tansy, and white hellebore.

Medical exams often included divination such as tarot readings, astrology, and other forms of witchcraft. Different remedies such as pills, charms, potions, and herbal medicines were prescribed, typically at extraordinarily high prices. Many times, this was brought to the attention of the garda, but even law enforcement officials feared the possibility of magical reprisals.

Some of the charms, potions and gris gris used by voodoo practitioners and what they are used for follow:

Absinthe: Aids in conjuring the dead to communicate if burnt with sandalwood as an incense.

African Ginger: Used by occultants to sprinkle in the 4 corners of a room. It is said to be pleasing to all spirits one wishes to conjure.

Ague weed: Causes one's enemies to become extremely confused.

Aloes: Traditionally used to invoke demons. It is said to soak aloes in a bottle of black cat oil for 9 days, on the 10th night anoint the forehead with the oils and the altar. The demon should appear to do one's bidding.

Anise seed: Used to increase the power in all psychic workings.

Asafoetida: Used in black magick for casting hexes on a person. Sometimes referred to as the devil's incense. Asafoetida is burned to force someone to leave you alone.

Balmony: A plant in the figwort family that is ground and used for hexing.

Betal Nut: A powerful ingredient in black magick arts. When chewed with lime, it is said to increase one's power, both spiritual and mental.

Bladderwrack: When placed near an enemy's bathroom, it is said to cause that enemy with irritation of the urinary tract.

Blood Root: If you are looking for a substitute for human blood, use this blood root to make diabolic wine.

Blueberry: Causes an enemy strife when thrown on his doorstep.

Boneset: To burn as an incense and chant. To be used during curses.

Cinquefoil: Burn over a candle wax image of an enemy to cause him discomfort.

Coconuts: Hollow out the coconut and fill with snakeroot. Place it in a flaming pit and as it roasts, your enemy's health will decline.

Cruel Man of the Woods: If a piece of this is hidden on your enemy's self, it will cause them great pain, if they have previously harmed you.

Henbane: All parts of this root is poisonous and boiling or dyeing does not bind its toxicity.

Knot Weed: To get rid of one's enemy. It is stuffed into a black cloth or voodoo doll and sewn up, then the doll is buried. It is also used with balmony herb in curses.

Lemon Verbena: Causes great trouble between lovers. When scattered at the doorway of the couple, great discord will ensue and the two will become bitter enemies.

Mustard Seed: The seed of strife and discord. Leave it at one's doorstep, particularly black mustard seed. This seed sprinkled around the trunk of a fruit tree on the first evening of the full moon will cause the tree to bear no fruit.

Patchouli: Sickens enemies when used in chants and spells.

Poke Root: A conjure ball can be made in the name of Satan from the leaves and root. It is placed into a glass jar or container and then left where the enemy will find it. This is done so that he will panic and be caused anxiety, making him more prone to accidents and injuries befalling him.

Poppy Seed: Causes couples to argue.

Rue: Although it is a great protection for the owner in turn, rue is placed near another person and puts a great hex on them. Since it is not a powerful black magic herb, it is used to simply frustrate or agitate the person, rather than causing them serious harm or injury.

Slippery Elm: Used to separate a married couple when burned near their home.

Tormentilla: To cause distress, harm, and discord to a foe. Sprinkle this on a picture of him or her and place it in a box.

Twitch's Grass: Causes quarrels among friends. Place under each leg of a table they will sit at. By the end of the evening, they will surely be fighting.

Vetivert: Silences one who will speak ill of you.

Vervain: Spells used to contact and speak with Lucifer are the most effective when using this herb. Also used for conjuring evil spirits and demons.

Willow: Willow is under the devil's protection and when held in one's left hand, may be used in pacts or rites requiring supernatural powers.

Wormwood: Used in making pacts with the devil (Authentic Voodoo: Herbs of the Darker Arts, 2010, p. 1).

Following is a partial listing of herbs used by many tribes, but the Cherokee, in particular:

Spignet	Backache	Make tea or powder of the roots
Rabbit Tobacco	Colds	Make tea of leaves and stalks
Red Alder	High blood	Made tea of bark
Wild Cherry	Measles and colds	Made tea of bark
Beech Bark	Vomiting	Make tea
Peach Leaves	Boils and risings	Make poultice from leaves and meal
Boneset	Pneumonia	Make tea of leaves and stalks

Small Ragweed	Poison Oak or Ivy	Heat leaves and rub on
Goldenrod	Consumption	Make tea of leaves and stalks
Ratbane	Typhoid fever	Make tea of leaves and stalks
Elder	Heartburn	Make tea of bark
Ginseng	Colic	Make tea of the roots
12 O'Clock Weed	Kills flies	Crush leaves in sweet milk
Queen of the Meadow	Nausea at certain times	Make tea of leaves and roots
Christmas Fern	Fever	Make tea of leaves or stems
Ground Ivy	Hives	Make tea of leaves or stems
Yellow Root	Sore mouth, sore throat, or stomach trouble	Make tea of the roots
Heat Leaves	Cold	Beat the whole plant and make tea
Bull Nettle	Stop teething babies from slobbering	Make beads of roots

Native American Medicinal Herbs-Partial Listing

Table 2.

(Cherokee By Blood: Medicine, p. 1)

Both Tommie Bass and Lelanie Stone have taught and mentored others in the identification and use of herbs. Lelanie has taken it to formal classrooms and workshops and then written books based on her research. Tommie, with a very low level of literacy, taught by voice and example, was the focus of a documentary, and had his work written and put into book form, using his own words.

Though Tommie stated that he gave away as much as he would sell of herbs and salves, Lelanie's give-aways are/were in the form of her books sometimes and help given through her website and articles.

Tommie didn't venture very far from his mountain in his work with herbs, but was in touch with folks from all over, both by phone and in letter. He said that he always answered every letter. Lelanie has traveled, researched, and lectured worldwide.

Both of them profess(ed) using what we have and that many of our medicines today are plant-based; that herbs support nature in fighting diseases. They are systems—cleansers-balancers.

Some of the harvesting rules-of-thumb that were common to both follow:

Don't pick herbs

- You don't recognize;
- By a roadside;
- In unfamiliar places;

- Don't pick all of any stand; and

- Don't put more than one herb in each sack.

Just as Lelanie was mentored by others and has turned around and taught others, Tommy Bass taught many such as Darryl Patton, who does the same thing to and for others, as well.

Both have used oral histories and information passed down from others, and in turn, have done the same thing. Tommie did the video and had information put down into written form. Lelanie has put hers in book form and minimally on the web.

Both Tommie Bass and Lelanie Anderson were/are astute business people, as well as excellent networkers. Tommie got help initially with labeling and selling his products. Word-of-mouth worked very well for him. In the video, it even shows him going to a flea market and listening to a fellow who was selling his products and that fellow turned around and told Tommie to sell his book while there. Through a cultivated friendship with a young lady, she and her husband were able to learn about herbs and to begin a very successful herb store. His products were sold there, as well.

Lelanie used/uses many means to market herself. Among those are her website, writing for local newspapers and the Oklahoma

Cherokee tribal newsletter, and lecturing at the local level, colleges and universities across the nation and worldwide, as well.

Both believed that herbs are gifts. Lelanie stated that "Native Americans of this continent knew the secrets held by Nature and Mother Earth, they used them to cure the sick and ailing people of their tribes long before there were white man's pharmacies or doctors on this continent. The Native Americans of this land aided the white settlers in their journeys in this untamed land, by lending them the knowledge of herbal remedies that Mother Nature had given them. These remedies and cures are more than just ideas or old wive's tales" (L. Stone, personal communication,1991).

Tommie stated in his book that, "God has put a herb here that will give temporary relief for men's ills . . . When God made the world, he planted the herbs, trees, grasses, etc. before he made anyone to see after the world. When he was pleased with his work, he took the dust and made man to look after the world. So, we are made of the ground and we have to look after the ground for the herbs, etc. to make the body tick . . . I always did believe that God never did make no mistakes. He never made anything He didn't make a remedy for. The Lord's put something out there if we would only get out there and hunt it" (Patton, 2004, p. 11).

CHAPTER TEN

Conclusions, Implications, and Recommendations
for Further Research

Conclusions

The thrust of this historical perspective has been to give you, the reader, a basic understanding of the past-to-present timeframe, the role of magic, religion, and mysticism, and the subsequent impact and influence that they have had through the ages. Additionally, having given that history, it is hoped that you will be able to articulate why modern-day herbalism has struggled in some instances, and in other instances, become a successful means of healing.

The druids and ancient Celts were nature-based, using plant/herb medicine for both remedies and cures. They gave us many of the remedies/medicinal applications which are in use today. Those were passed down primarily through oral tradition. Along with being healers, they controlled others through the practice of being intercessors to the deities. Fear and awe abounded, as the druids used perceived dietific power combined with herbal knowledge for both good and ill. As Christianity entered and pagan worship was forced underground for the most part, so to speak, the application and use of many of the remedies were touted to be heresy and punishable through the Church, with penalties as heavy as death.

When the Church had, for the most part, wiped out active druidism, they began a campaign known as witch hunts. This came in the form of the Inquisition and later, the Reformation. There were all levels of what were known to be witches. Some were plant/herb doctors and/or healers; some simply touted themselves to be (i.e., quacks and cunning-folk) for the money; some worked in the dark arts, to work with dark forces, using herb/plant skills to harm others and/or for control/power; and still others were simply victims of the Church. At this point, we see Christianity stepping in and a seed of doubt having turned into full-blown fear, relative to those practicing plant/herb medicine.

Two events occurred in the United States in the 1700's; one being the immigration of Scottish and Irish to the Appalachian Mountains and the other, being the slave trade from Africa to Haiti and then to the southern United States. The slave trade, brought individuals, which due to the slave owners, practiced both Catholicism and Voodoo, to the south. The individuals also brought some knowledge of plant/herb medicine. As was presented, that knowledge was also used in conjunction with power and control. As with the druids, voodoo priests and priestesses (especially, Marie Laveau) used it to control individuals, and even local businesses, law enforcement, and politicians. Hollywood glamorized the role of zombies and marketing promoters turned a good luck charm into a feared totem. Plant and herb medicine, mixed with charms, potions, superstition, magic, and the Catholic religion continue to make the use of plant remedies a field of fear, suspicion, awe, and speculation.

Implications

As has been presented, many of the healing traditions still exist in the Appalachians. Though Granny Women aren't as prevalent as in the past, some still exist. Many more people, even outside of the area, in and out of colleges, such as Darryl Patton, Phyllis Light, and Lelanie Stone, are teaching/mentoring others. That knowledge isn't solely relegated to families as it was before. Additionally, other traditions passed from as far back as the druids and ancient Celts, such as Celtic holidays connected to seasonal/nature-based changes are still recognized and honored:

- St. Brigid's Day-February 1st: The beginning of Spring;

- St. Patrick's Day-March 17th: The Middle of spring season and spring equinox;

- May Day/Beltaine-May 1st: The start of the summer season;

- Midsummer/Summer Solstice-June 23rd: The longest day of the year;

- Lughnasa-August 1st: Beginning of the harvest;

- Autumnal Equinox-September 21st:The harvest is collected and the length of night and day are the same;

- Samhain-October 31st-November 1st:The darker half of the year begins and winter is coming;

- Winter Solstice-December 21st-23rd: The shortest day of the year (Muldoon, 2001, January 5, p. 2).

Native Americans, in the 1700's, already had at least 600 documented formulas. Of these, approximately 250 medicinal formulas were added to the official Pharmacopoeia (Hatter, 2007, para 3). Samuel Thompson combined his mother's herbal medical techniques and combined these with what he knew of Native American remedies. From this, he developed Thompsonian Herbalism in the 1840's. Additionally, Cherokee plant knowledge was eventually translated into the Cherokee Herbal. (Garrett, 1942)

Native Americans continue to use plant remedies and most IHS (Indian Health Service) facilities offer the services of traditional medicine men and women and ceremony in conjunction with allopathic care. Evidence of this is seen in studies such as:

1. One study found that "Use of traditional healing was more common for physical than psychiatric problems among participants from both the Southwest (22.9% vs. 7.8% respectively) and Northern Plains (8.4% vs. 3.2%). In addition, use of traditional healing was more prevalent in the Southwest than the Northern Plains for physical health and psychiatric problems" (Douglas, Beals, Moore, Spicer, Manson, 2004);

2. A Navajo study on healers found that "certain complaints such as family problems and insomnia were much more common reasons for visits to native healers than medical providers. Those who saw native healers for depression/ anxiety and arthritis were less likely to consult a medical provider, and medical providers were never consulted for

"sickness", "blessing", "bad luck", or family problems" (Kim, Yeong, 1998);

3. A study conducted in an urban Native American health center found that "Most patients report seeing a healer for spiritual reasons. The most frequently visited healers were herbalists, spiritual healers, and medicine men. Sweat lodge ceremonies, spiritual healing, and herbal medicines were the most common treatments. More than a third of the patients seeing healers received different advice from their physicians and healers" (Marbella, Harris, Diehr, Ignance, Ignance, 1998);

4. In a diabetes education study with the Cheyenne River Sioux Tribe, it was "suggested that more culturally specific intervention approaches might lead to greater behavioral change than standardized interventions" (Kattlemann, Conti, Ren, 2009); and

5. In a study conducted on healing through the use of Navajo Indian medicine, it was found that "Most seriously ill Navajos utilize both systems of health care. Traditional ceremonies are successful because they are integrated into Navajo belief systems and meet needs of sick people not dealt with by the available Western medicine" (Coulehan, 1980).

Mysticism and superstition still surrounds the role of medicine people and the use of herbs in healing. However, many Native Americans, through cultural and familial knowledge use herbs for remedies. Additionally, many in the reservation areas and tribal land, such as in Cherokee, North Carolina and the area surrounding Tahlequah and Stilwell, Oklahoma, utilize their knowledge to bring in incomes through wildcrafting.

The role of witchcraft has changed and evolved through the ages. As has been presented, it had/has a very healthy role in the Appalachians. The medicinal application of herbs, as well as wildcrafting has continued, though with the influx of allopathic healthcare, the role of herbal doctors and granny magic, isn't as widespread as in past years.

Witchcraft in mainstream society, has a very different connotation and is still a much-feared practice by the majority of Christians. The use of herbs within the practice of "The Craft" is considered at the very least, to be dangerous. It is typically associated with dark arts, even though there are many new titles ascribed to it, such as "New Age," "Green Witchery," "Wicca," and "White Witchcraft."

Summary

Government regulation of herbs, in addition to the powerful role played by pharmaceutical companies has posed a problem for herb companies, small businesses and naturopathy, in general. However, there are strong advocates such as Darryl Patton, practitioner organizations (i.e., American Association of Drugless Practitioners, American Herbalist Guild, American Naturopathic Certification Board, Coalition for Natural Health, and the National Center for Homeopathy), and lobbyists, who have slowly effected changes. Additionally, with recent health care initiatives and legislation, many more individuals are changing their minds about the role of prescription and over-the-counter drug usage. Many are turning back to the natural remedies and embracing a greener way of life, both for physical health and economic reasons. They are educating themselves through the media, through classes and workshops, through books, through the internet, and through word-of-mouth.

The United States is a melting pot of culture, races, and ethnicities. Herbalism today, is a very valuable evidence of what seven primary and diverse cultures (Celts, druids, witchcraft, Native Americans, Voodoo, Christianity, and Appalachians) have brought forward. Through the blending of all of these cultures, each with their histories, each with their knowledge and skills in plant medicine, each with their own religious beliefs, each with a level of superstition, mysticism and magic, have brought an incredible wealth of knowledge for use, application, and education in the field of herbalism today. The history, though, is important to that knowledge.

REFERENCES

Authentic Voudou (2010, p. 1). Retrieved from www.erzulies.com

Barish, S. A. (2008). Use of complimentary and alternative healthcare practices among persons served by a remote area medical clinic. *Family Community Health, July-Sep* 31 (3), 221-7. Retrieved from http://www.ncbi.nlm.nih.gov/pubmed/18552603

Blake, P. (2008). Native American Thompsonian herbalism. *Articlesbase SC, 369013.* Retrieved from http://www. articlesbase.com

Cannon, WB (2002). "Voodoo" death. American Anthropologist, 1942;44 (new series):169-181. Retrieved from PMID: 12356599 [PubMed—indexed for MEDLINE]PMCID: PMC1447285

Carpenter, A., Page, L. G., & Wigginton, E. (1983). *Aunt Arie: a Foxfire portrait (pp. 117, 121).* New York: Dutton.

Celtic Medicine Wheel of the British Isles (2010, p.1). Retrieved from http://www.sacredhome.co.uk/wheel.html

Cherokee Culture. Retrieved from http://www.aaanativehearts.com/ cherokee-culture.htm

Cherokee Medicine Men and Women—Cherokee Nation. Retrieved from www.cherokee.org/Culture/13/Page/default.aspx

Cherokee Messenger (1996, January, p. 1). Retrieved from http://www.powersource.com/cherokee/message/0196.htm

Clancy, Shae. Ancient Celts and their environment in 'earth sea and sky' (p.3). Retrieved from http://www.aughty.org/pdf/ancient_celts.pdf

Classical Traditional Naturopathy-What is Naturopathy? (p.2). Retrieved from http://www.classicalnaturopathy.org/naturopathy/html

Cohen, K. (1998). Native American medicine. *Altern Ther Health Med, Nov*(4 (6)), 45-47. Retrieved November 9, 2010, from http://www.ncbi.nlm.nih.gov/pubmed/9810067

Comfort, A. (1981). Sorcery and sudden death. *J R Soc Med, May 74(5)(p.333)*. Retrieved November 16, 2010, from http://www.ncbi.nlm.nih.gov/pmc/articles/PMC1438836/?tool=pubmed

Coulehan, J. (1980). Navajo Indian medicine: implications for healing. *Family Practice, Jan* 10 (1), 55-61. Retrieved from http://www.ncbi.nlm.nih.gov/pubmed/7350261

Coyne, Cathy, Damien-Popescu, Cristina, and Friend, Dana, (2006). Social and cultural factors influencing health in southern West Virginia: A qualitative study. *Prev Chronic Dis. 3 (4)* October,

A124. Retrieved from http://www.ncbi.nlm.nih/gov/pmc/articles/ PMC1779

Crockett, David C. (1971). Medicine among the American Indians. HSMHA Health Reports May 1971, Vol. 86, No. 5, pp. 399-407. Retrieved from http://www.ncbi.nlm.nih.gov-pmc-articles-PMC1775810-pdf-amjph00789-0051.pdf.url

Davies, O. (1999). Cunning-folk in the medical market-place during the nineteenth century. *Medical History, 43,* 55-73. Retrieved from http://www.ncbi.nlm.nih.gov/pubmed/10885133

Druidry and Christianity. Retrieved from http://www.dobhran.com/ DPchristian.htm

Dudgeon, Roy (n.d.).The Meaning and use of the medicine wheel case study: Lakota

Philosophy (p. 3). Retrieved from sixcrows.org/docs/MedicineWheel MeaningandUse.pdf

Folk medicine and health beliefs: an Appalachian perspective [J Cult Divers. 1996]—PubMed result. (n.d.). *National Center for Biotechnology Information*. Retrieved from http://www.ncbi. nlm.nih.gov/pubmed/9418440

Foxwood, Orion (2009, January 29, p. 4). Magic: A living folk tradition. Retrieved from http://www.exploreyourspirit.com/ blog/2009/01/29/magic-a-living- tradition-by-orion-foxwood/

Garrett, J. T. (2003). *The Cherokee herbal: native plant medicine from the four directions*. Rochester, Vt.: Bear & Company.

Haitian voodoo. Retrieved from http://travelinghaiti.com/haitian_ voodoo.asp

Hatter. Ila (2007). Appalachian healing traditions, *Talk for Cleveland Symposium—April 4, 2007.* Retrieved from http://www. wildcrafting.com/appalachian_healing_traditions.htm

Hemphill, R. (1966). Historical Witchcraft and psychiatric illness in Western Europe. *Proceedings of the Royal Society of Medicine, Volume 59,* 891-902.Retrieved from http://www.ncbi.nlm.nih. gov/pmc/articles/PMC1901240

Holy Bible. (1977, p. 597). Nashville: Thomas Nelson Publishers.

Irwin, J. R. (1985). *Alex Stewart, portrait of a pioneer(p. 135, chapter 5)*. West Chester, Pa.: Schiffer Pub.

James, B. (1894). *Irish Druids and old Irish religions* (pp. 24-25). S. Low: Griffith and Fausan.

Kattelmann K. K, Conti K, Ren C. (2009). The Medicine Wheel nutrition intervention: a diabetes education study with the Cheyenne River Sioux Tribe. Republished from: *J Am Diet Assoc. 2009 Sep;109(9):1532-9.* Nutrition, Food Science and Hospitality Department, South Dakota State University, Brookings, SD 57007, USA.

Keith G. Tidball and Chris Toumey (2007). Serpents, sainthood, and celebrity: Symbolic and ritual tension in Appalachian Pentecostal snake handling, *Journal of Religion and Popular Culture, Vol. 17, Fall.* Retrieved from www.usask.ca/relst/jrpc/art17-serpents. html

Kim, Catherine and Kwok, Yeong S. (1998). Navajo use of native healers. Archives of Internal Medicine; 158:2245-2249. Retrieved from altmed.creighton.edu/AmericanIndianMed/ Kim%20research.htm

Klemens, Jonathan, (2008). Ancient Celtic myth, magic, and medicine. *Feedbooks, 22138.* Retrieved from http://www. writers.net/221138.

Kwok, K. C. (1998). Native use of native healers. *Arch Intern Med, 158 (20),* 2245-9. Retrieved from http://www.ncbi.nlm.nih.gov/ pubmed/9818804

Lee, M. (2006). Solanaceae III: henbane, hags, and Hawley Harvey Crippen. *JR Co U Physicians, Edinb., Dec.* 36 (4), 366-73. Retrieved from http://www.ncbi.nlm.nih.gov/ pubmed/17526134

Louisiana Voodoo. Retrieved from http://en.wikipedia.org/wiki/ Louisiana_Voodoo

Marbella A.M., Harris M.C., Diehr S., Ignace G., Ignace G. (1998). Use of Native American healers among Native American patients in an urban Native American health center. *Arch Fam Med.* Mar-Apr;7(2):182-5. Retrieved from www.ncbi.nlm.nih. gov/pubmed/9519925

Matthews, J. & Stewart, R. J. (1988). *Celtic battle heroes: Cuchulainn: Boadicea—Fionn MacCumhaill: Macbeth, (p.2).* Poole, Dorset: Firebird Books.

MEDEA Study Guide (p. 4, 6). Retrieved from http://www.colleges. org/faculty_renewal/reports/2009/BSC_Litsey

Medicine Wheel (p.3). Retrieved from www.absoluteastronomy.com

Medicine Wheel. Retrieved from http://www.en.wikipedia.org/wiki/ Medicine_wheel

Methods of Treatment (p.2). Retrieved from http://allmedcreighton. edu/American

Indian/Med/Methods.htm

Mooney, J. (1992). *James Mooney's history, myths, and sacred formulas of the Cherokees: containing the full texts of Myths of the Cherokee (1900) and the sacred formulas of the Cherokees (1891) as published by the Bureau of American Ethnology : with a new biographical intr.* Asheville, N.C.: Historical Images.

Muldoon, Molly (2011, January 5, p.1). The eight sacred Celtic holidays of the new year. Retrieved from http://www.irishcentral.com

Native American Medicine Wheels—History and Meaning. Retrieved from www.support-native-american-art.com/Native-American-Medicine-Wheels.html

[No authors listed], (a. (1897). Archaeologica Medica: XXXV.-Ancient Celtic physicians. *The British Medical Journal, 11;2 (1915)* Sept. 669. Retrieved from http://www.ncbi.nlm.nih.gov/pubmed

Novins, D. K.; Beals, J.; Moore, L. A.; Spicer, P.; & Manson, S. M. (2004). *Use of Traditional Healing,* Volume 42(7) 2004. Retrieved from Use of Traditional Healing.altmed.creighton.edu/AmericanIndianMed /Novins%20research.htm

Orman, S. (2006). *The 9 steps to financial freedom: Practical and spiritual steps so you can stop worrying* (Updated & rev. 3rd ed.). New York: Three Rivers Press.

Patton, D. (2004). *Mountain medicine: The herbal remedies of Tommie Bass (pp. 11, 13).* Birmingham, AL: Natural Reader Press.

Robbins, R. H. (1959). *The encyclopedia of witchcraft and demonology.* New York: Crown Publishers.

Shelley, B. M.; Sussman, A. L.; Williams, R. L.; Segal, A. R.; Crabtree, B. F.; & Rios Net Clinicians, a. o. (2009). They don't ask me so I don't tell them: Patient-clinician communication about traditional, complimentary, and alternative medicine. *Ann Fam Med, March* 7(2), 139-147. Retrieved from http://www. ncbi.nlm.nih.gov/pmc/articles/PMC265970

Snake Handlers (p.1). Retrieved from www.georgiaencyclopedia. org/nge/Article.jsp

Stilwell, Ginger (2001, Januray 8). Appalachian and granny magic. Retrieved from http://www.witchvox.com

Stone, L. F. (1991). *Indian herbs and plants (p.1)*. Locust Grove, Okla.: Stone Studio.

Stone, Mary Butler, (n.d., p.1). Appalachian folk medicine. Retrieved from http://home.wlu.edu~lubint/TouchstoneAppalchianFolkMed. Stone.htm

Struthers, R., & Patchel, B. (2008). The experience of being an Anishiabe man healer; ancient healing in a modern world. *J Cult Divers, Summer* 16(2), 70-5. Retrieved from http://www.ncbi. nlm.nih.gov/pubmed/2066630017

The Herbal Medicine Wheel (an unpublished book copyright 1983 by Gary J. Lockhart 1983, pp. 8-14). Edited and PDF of part placed online by Arthur Lee Jacobson in 2007.The Medicine

Wheel. Retrieved from http://www.dancingtoeaglespiritsociety. org/medwheel.php

The Order of Bards Ovates & Druids. Retrieved from http://druidry. org/ Traditional Naturopathy. Retrieved from http://www.ccnh. edu/healthy/traditionalnaturopathy

Tulsa Area Chapter, T. A. (1996). *American Indians decision to survive* (pp. 27, 33, 46). Tulsa, Ok: American National Red Cross.

Vann, David. Cherokee by blood. Retrieved from http:// cherokeebyblood.com/medicine.htm

Vodun (a.k.a. Voodoo and related religions). Retrieved from http:// religioustolerance.com

Voodoo. Retrieved from http://www.hauntedamericatours.com/ voodoo/voodooqueens/voodoo

Voodoo. Retrieved from http://www.llewellyn.com/encyclopedia/ term/voodoo

Webb, Julie Yvonne, R.N., M.S. Hyg. (1971). Louisiana Voodoo and superstitions related to health. *HSMHA Health Rep.*, *April* 86 (4), 291-301. Retrieved from http://www.ncbi.nlm.nih.gov/pmc/ articles/PMC1937133/pdf/hsmhahr00004-0005.pdf

What Is An Ovate? Retrieved from http://www.druidry.org/ modules

Wigginton, E., & Bennett, M. (1977, 1986). *Foxfire 9: General stores, the Jud Nelson wagon . . . (pp. 346-347).* (Anchor Books ed.). New York, N.Y.: Anchor Books/Doubleday.

Wilde, L. W. (1997). *Celtic women in legend, myth and history.* London: Blandford. Thompson, Cindy (2010, March 8).

THE REAL TRUE GREAT VOODOO QUEENS AND KINGS. Retrieved from http://celticvoices.blogspot.com

Winston, David, AHG (2001). Nvwoti; Cherokee Medicine and Ethnobotany. *American Herbalism Essays on Herbalism. Crossings 1992.* Retrieved from www.herbaltherapeutics.net/ CherokeeMed.(expanded)805.pdf